The Upgrade

Also by Louann Brizendine

The Female Brain
The Male Brain

The Upgrade

*How the Female Brain
Gets Stronger and Better
in Midlife and Beyond*

Louann Brizendine, MD

with Amy Hertz

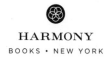

HARMONY

BOOKS · NEW YORK

No book can replace the diagnostic expertise and medical advice of a trusted physician. Please be certain to consult with your doctor before making any decisions that affect your health, particularly if you suffer from any medical conditions or have any symptoms that may require treatment.

Library of Congress Cataloging-in-Publication Data
Names: Brizendine, Louann, author. | Hertz, Amy, other.
Title: The upgrade : how the female brain gets stronger and better in
   midlife and beyond / Louann Brizendine, MD with Amy Hertz.
Description: First edition. | New York : Harmony Books, [2022] | Includes
   bibliographical references and index.
Identifiers: LCCN 2021035518 (print) | LCCN 2021035519 (ebook) |
   ISBN 9780525577171 (hardcover) | ISBN 9780525577188 (ebook)
Subjects: LCSH: Brain. | Brain—Sex differences. | Women. | Brain—
   Psychology.
Classification: LCC QP376 .B76 2022 (print) | LCC QP376 (ebook) |
   DDC 612.8/2082--dc23/eng/20211001
LC record available at lccn.loc.gov/2021035518
LC ebook record available at lccn.loc.gov/2021035519

ISBN 978-0-525-57717-1
Ebook ISBN 978-0-525-57718-8

Printed in the United States of America

Book design and illustrations by Andrea Lau
Jacket design by Anna Bauer Carr

10 9 8 7 6 5 4 3 2 1

First Edition

To my mother, Louise Ann Stocksdale Brizendine
In memoriam

Never stop trying to solve the puzzle of your life.
Engage until the very end.

———

Contents

Author's Note

I thought I would never write another book again. But as I entered the second half of life myself and started to feel the invisibility reserved uniquely for women of a certain age, something inside me rebelled. I could feel a new power, a new clarity, a laser-like sense of purpose emerging in this phase, and I knew it was time to explore the new science that supported what I was feeling. This was not a slow decline toward the end: I was staring down the most vital, confident, and wise phase of my life. There was a name for the second half of life and we weren't yet using it. I call it the Upgrade. Formerly known as menopause, the Upgrade is the phase of life we emerge into when we exit the hormonal war zone finally able to see and be present to who we are, what we want, and how we want to live. It's a glorious time full of freedom and discovery.

As I put the finishing touches on the manuscript, the first female vice president took the oath of office. The cabinet of the forty-sixth president is full of women, most of them also in the second half of life. I began to feel a hopefulness that I thought had been buried with the defeat of the Equal Rights Amendment in the 1970s and '80s. I felt the door to possibility crack open personally and collectively for embracing a productive second half.

As a neuropsychiatrist specializing in the impact of women's hormones on the brain, i.e., emotions, thoughts, values, priorities, even perception, I think of myself as a medical and psychological scout for the tribe of women. I love going out ahead for reconnaissance, gathering useful information from neuroscience and medical studies to bring back to help others find their own way forward, to understand what is happening to them physically and how that changes everything from mood to sense of identity. This may sound silly, but it encapsulates my motivation to bring you the information about the road ahead in this book.

The Upgrade is about the path to becoming your best deep self—okay, maybe it's a bit grandiose, but if not now, when? In the second half of my life, I want to upgrade my skills and improve my willingness to take responsibility for doing so. I want to develop my enthusiasm, patience, humility, commitment, and determination to make the most of this life transition; recharge my brain and my self-compassion as I search for a new reality, new connections, a new sense of "me." I want a new relationship to myself and others and to return to a larger purpose with renewed focus. Honoring my health span, I want to attend to the care of my body and mind so that the Upgrade becomes possible.

The Upgrade delves into doubts and misinformation in order to help you find your own answers. It is about solving the conflicts you have in your mind about how emotions, hormones, biology, and the brain work together. It is about having the courage to examine all of our qualities, rejoicing in some and improving others. It is about realizing you have a choice about your path in the second half of life.

So much of what feels normal and natural to us, when you look closely, is soft-wired into us by hormones and environment. Some of it is great and helpful, but we receive so many messages about our supposed irrelevance in the second half of life that I've decided it's time to punch through. The more you know about neurochemicals, brain circuits, and the neurons throughout the body, the greater your chances of breaking out of old patterns to create a new life. And the greater the chance we'll be able to reach behind to the next generation and help them too.

I'm acutely aware that my experience and the experience of the women I have encountered in my life will not represent the reality for many women who have struggled under much harsher conditions than I can understand and continue to function while carrying the heavy burden of systemic racism. Many of the women in this book identify as BIPOC (Black, Indigenous, and people of color) and all of them as cisgender, i.e., the female identity they were born with; their Transition and Upgrade stories exemplify experiences that reach across boundaries of race. Out of respect for the individuality of experience, I chose not to write outside my own knowledge and the understanding I have gained from my patients, family, and friends. To that end, I can't adequately address at this time the Upgrade for transgender men and women. There is so much still unknown and under-researched that it might do more harm than good, but where there is something known, it is mentioned. And where there is something known about racial and cultural differences and the Upgrade, it is also mentioned. Structural racism is embedded in the healthcare system; that is a given. I promise to do whatever I can to support the emergence of the Upgrade for all women.

To be seen, heard, and valued is what we all want, and what we need to give to one another and the ones we love. I have laid out the things I know and have experienced, the obstacles and glories in the Upgrade. But as yet there are no real developmental landmarks for women in the second half, and creating them so that we all can find our way forward is a collective effort. I want to learn about your struggles and victories, too. And more than anything I want you to know how much I value your experience and wisdom.

I hope that something here might give you support, knowledge, understanding, and courage to overcome the many obstacles in the second half. We're all in this together. So let's start the conversation that no one seems to want us to have about life after the fertile phase.

Changing the Conversation Starts with Using the Right Words

I am proposing a new vocabulary for menopause and perimenopause, so that we don't have to rely on the M-word and the P-word, which literally refer to the end of fertility.

The Transition: The developmental phase of a woman's life in which the brain and body enter unfamiliar territory as the reproductive-phase circuits are finishing their job. This is the phase formerly known as perimenopause.

Just as the teen years are about so much more than hormones, so is the Transition. The hormonal transition that shuts down fertility is front and center, but it doesn't remotely tell the whole story, nor does it represent who we are. There are also many psychological growth phases within the Transition that include identity and the path toward authenticity. The Transition marks a change in our relationships and societal roles. None of these transitions are explored in any of the literature about the phases of human development.

The Upgrade: The wisdom phase that emerges after spending decades in the hormonal war zone. Emerging into the most powerful identity phase of a woman's life, this is what was formerly known as menopause or postmenopause.

"Perimenopause" and "menopause" are fossil words created by men at pharmaceutical companies. These words arose not because of an interest in helping women reach the Upgrade, which is a whole-person explosion of growth and realization of potential. These words arose as men studied how to maintain elasticity and fullness in the parts of our bodies they, as cisgender men, like to interact with, i.e., breasts and vaginas. I don't believe they encompass the full scope of the Upgrade, and so I decline to use them, other than in this note explaining my reasons. And if you catch me using them anywhere else in the book, snap a picture or screenshot of the page, find me at Dr. Louann Brizendine on Facebook, @louannbrizendine on Instagram, and @DrLouann on Twitter, and take me to task! I can't wait to hear from you all directly.

Hormone therapy (HT): Replaces the older term "hormone replacement therapy" (HRT), which is a less accurate term. When we use hormones, we aren't replacing, we are adding.

The Four Phases of the Transition

Pre-Transition: It happens as the number of viable eggs declines and fewer follicles are formed, impacting the amount of sex hormones produced each month. You might notice a bit more anxiety just before your period, a bit more trouble cooling off after an intense aerobic workout, or a little bit of heat or sweating at night. Your sleep might be interrupted around the time of your period. The Pre-Transition begins on average in your late thirties.

Early Transition: This is marked by more noticeable sleep disruption—you may find yourself fully drenched or wake up with the covers thrown off—at least once a week or so. In the Early Transition you might experience occasional irregular bleeding—less volume and fewer days or a bit more blood over a day or two—skipped periods, midmonth breakthrough bleeding or spotting. This happens because of an increase in a common, normal event: anovulation, or an eggless cycle.

Mid-Transition: You have two or three short cycles in a year, going from, say, twenty-eight down to twenty-seven or twenty-six or twenty-five days. This phase is marked by more frequent sleep disruption—several times a week—and feeling hot.

Late Transition: This phase is characterized by nightly sleep disruption, hot flashes, and between three and ten shortened cycles per year.

The Three Stages of the Upgrade

Early Upgrade: Twelve months after your last period marks the beginning of this phase. Some women who still have a uterus choose HT that mimics their natural cycles; they will continue to bleed monthly. Many others experience a combination of joy over no more periods and shock in the face of a changing body.

Middle Upgrade: This phase involves attempting to make friends with the new reality, exploring new life paths, feeling the pull of needing a break, and desperately wanting to heed the siren's call to disengage.

Full Upgrade: This stage means embodying the fullness of life, embracing the ups and downs, returning to purpose, speaking truth skillfully and effectively, engaging as a mentor and sponsor, being pulled by the desire to leave humanity better than you found it.

I haven't included ages here, because the Transition stages can begin and end at different times. So much depends on the individual. I've seen some reach the Full Upgrade immediately and others remain in Early Upgrade for life. Where you are depends on your attitude and your actions.

Neurochemicals (i.e., Hormones and Neurohormones) You'll Need to Know About

Ovarian hormones:

- Estrogen: Secreted by the follicle that grows and spurts out an egg, estrogen drives growth in the uterine lining and in brain synapses. It controls brain energy and inflammation. It improves mood and bolsters mental acuity, word retrieval, and outgoing, flirty, affectionate behavior.
- Progesterone: The hormone of retaining, it keeps the uterine lin-

ing in place to receive a fertilized egg and puts the brakes on synaptic overgrowth in the brain. It's the comfy, cozy hormone that makes us want to curl up by a fire and eat cake. It's also responsible for the brain fog of pregnancy. "Progestins" is the word for various synthetic progesterones.

- Testosterone: It drives libido, muscle stimulation, and zest for life. I often experience this as the *Out of my way, mother f#$ker* feeling I get when my husband tries to stop to chat as I pass through the kitchen late on my way to the office. Ninety percent of it comes from the ovaries before the transition. After the Upgrade, 90 percent comes from the adrenal glands.

Adrenal hormones:

- Adrenaline (also referred to as epinephrine): Provides the necessary burst of energy to respond physically and mentally in a moment of danger. Causes a feeling of edginess.
- Noradrenaline (also referred to as norepinephrine): The main neurotransmitter coming from the adrenal glands for the sympathetic nerves and the cardiovascular system. It's what causes your heart to pump like crazy so that you can run away from danger.
- Cortisol: The stress hormone. Its impact on the limbic, or emotional brain is ten times higher than its impact on other brain areas. It suppresses the immune system and in excess it can lead to depression, irritability, and cognitive decline.
- Pregnenolone: A parent hormone that creates progesterone, DHEA, testosterone, estrogens, cortisol, and others. It helps us sleep well; it boosts sex drive, mood, memory, and attention; and it's good for the skin, joints, and muscles.
- DHEA (dehydroepiandrosterone): The mother hormone out of which come testosterone and estrogen. It counteracts cortisol, has antidepressant effects, improves sex drive, causes acne, and increases body odor.

Brain and nervous system chemicals
that get used all over the body:

- Follicle-stimulating hormone (FSH): The pituitary produces this chemical to get the ovary to form follicles to get the best eggs ready for launch. The follicles are what produce most of the estrogen, progesterone, and testosterone before the Upgrade.
- Luteinizing hormone (LH): The pituitary produces this chemical to get the best follicle to shoot its egg into the fallopian tube on its way to the uterus. It triggers the release of the egg.
- Oxytocin: This is produced in the hypothalamus and stored in the pituitary. Anytime estrogen kicks up, the hypothalamus will send out a little bucket full of this bonding, cuddling hormone of affection.
- GABA (gamma-aminobutyric acid): Ninety percent of all brain cells have receptors for this chemical, which is the body's natural Valium. It acts like a nice warm bubble bath on the inside.
- ALLO: Allopregnanolone is the molecule that progesterone converts into. It interacts with the calming GABAergic system that runs throughout the brain and entire nervous system.
- ACTH: Adrenocorticotropic hormone is produced and secreted by the pituitary to stimulate the adrenals to make cortisol.
- CRH: Corticotrophin-releasing hormone is produced by the hypothalamus and, when sent to the pituitary, triggers a rise in ACTH. This happens when the amygdala senses danger or threat.
- Acetylcholine: This is the chief neurotransmitter of the parasympathetic nervous system, the calming part of the nervous system, which slows the heart. It's the opposite of epinephrine. It is key to memory consolidation during sleep. Low levels are linked to learning and memory impairments.

Cells You'll Want to Know About

- Neurons: These are garden-variety brain and nerve cells, the ones you read about in high school biology. The surprise is that they are not the most numerous type of cell in the brain. They have a rival!
- Astrocytes: They are as numerous as neurons, and their job is to provide nutrients to the brain cells and keep harmful substances out.
- Microglia: These are scavenger cells that can control the connections between neurons and protect the brain from infection. During the day, the brain sprouts all kinds of connections and also discharges energy and waste from those new connections. During sleep, as the brain shrinks, the channels around the nerve cells can relax and open up, the microglia come in and prune away all the overgrowth.

Concepts You'll Want to Know About

- "Sterile" Inflammation: The chronic low-level immune inflammation unrelated to infections caused by stresses such as environmental conditions like UV radiation, mechanical trauma, cell death, hormones and leaking proteins, lack of sleep, and decreased blood flow. Sex differences in the immune system make it worse with age in males.
- Double X: The typical female has two X chromosomes so we have many brain and immune genes from the second X that may be protective against cognitive decline. This may be the secret to female longevity.

Drawings

The Female Brain

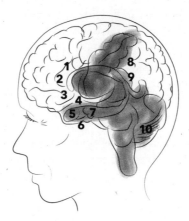

1. Prefrontal Cortex: The queen that rules the emotions and keeps them from going wild. It puts the brakes on the amygdala.

2. Nucleus Accumbens (NAc): The neural interface between desire and action, the bridge between wanting the goody and figuring out a way to get it.

3. Insula: The judge, jury, and executioner especially when it comes to self-image. "Gut feelings" occur here.

4. Hypothalamus: The conductor of the hormonal symphony; kicks the gonads into gear and struggles to manage as they go offline.

5. Amygdala: Snap decisions about life and death threats. Sometimes it perceives life and death when it's only a decision about where to park at the grocery store.

6. Pituitary: Produces hormones of fertility and screams like a junkie in detox when they are cut off.

7. Hippocampus: The elephant, larger and more effective in women, that never forgets a fight, a romantic encounter, or a tender moment, and won't let you forget it either. Though details will begin to fade in the Upgrade.

8/9. TPJ and Precuneus: When these two regions get into lockstep, you will be trapped on the hamster wheel of worry and sucked into the vortex of rumination. It's hard to achieve escape velocity to get out, but with a few tricks and tips, you can!

10. Cerebellum: The part of the brain that coordinates movement and balance for walking and standing. It helps almost every other part of the brain do its job better. It smooths your movements and your thinking and inhibits impulsive decision-making. It helps regulate emotion.

The brain's Default Mode Network (DMN): Connects areas in the front, middle, and back of the brain and turns on when the mind wanders. It rolls around like a big ball of Velcro picking up all kinds of negative thoughts. Meditation and ketamine turn this network off!

Threat/Stress Reaction: The fight-or-flight system, activates behavior to deal with threat; afterward, the calming reset comes from the vagal system.

HPA (hypothalamic pituitary adrenal) Axis, the so-called Stress Axis

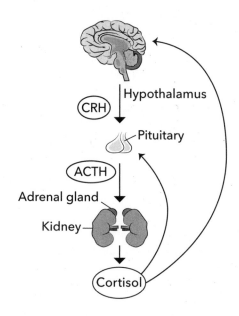

HPA controls release of cortisol (stress hormone) and androgen DHEA

HPO Axis (hypothalamic pituitary ovarian)
Reproductive Axis

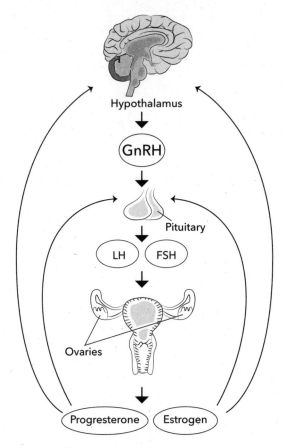

Hypothalamus

GnRH

Pituitary

LH FSH

Ovaries

Progresterone Estrogen

HPO controls release of estrogen, progesterone, and testosterone

Changing the Conversation

Chapter 1

In 1980, while on a research program during medical school at Yale, a mysterious illness landed me in the hospital in London, where I was doing a student clerkship. I was weak, achy, and so low in energy it felt like I was going to die. They did every test possible but never came up with a diagnosis. No lurking cancer, no rare infectious disease, no organ malfunction, no autoimmune issue. Everything came back normal. At one point I realized that some visiting residents were probing my sense of humor to evaluate whether or not I belonged in a psych ward. They concluded I didn't.

After ten days, I was released and returned to the United States for my fourth year of medical school. I was taken off the plane in New York in a wheelchair and paid for a limo back to New Haven. I appealed to the dean for some breathing room, but without a diagnosis, I was given no time off and got very little sympathy from faculty, family, or friends. My social support evaporated as people either didn't believe me or began to see me as difficult.

I did what I had to do to muscle through. I took an apartment across from the hospital in order to be able to go back to sleep after 5:30 A.M. rounds. Somehow I made it through, wrote my dissertation, and graduated.

During surgical and internal medicine rounds, I watched doctors and doctors-in-training stride across hospital rooms at 6:00 A.M., lifting up gowns to begin their examinations without even saying hello to the human beings in the bed. They didn't engage, they didn't ask questions—not even "How are you today?"—and they didn't seem to hear anyone but other doctors. And with the sickest of patients, when they ran out of tools, physicians disappeared, abandoning people who had lives and experiences and families much like their own, without so much as a farewell. They left that to the nurses.

Fresh off my own experience in London, I really knew what that felt like for patients. It's why I decided to go into psychiatry. I refused to be involved in any specialty in which I wouldn't have time to listen.

The brain, in fact the entire human nervous system of which the brain is a part, is hungry for connection. The feedback that we get from conversation, from sincere questions, tells us that we are accepted and that we belong. When we don't get this essential social vitamin, we starve the circuits of the nutrients they need. We get sicker. Our mental acuity withers. Depression creeps into and attacks our system.

Being abandoned, by doctors and by our social support, teaches us to abandon ourselves.

This is what made me start the Women's Mood and Hormone Clinic at UCSF in 1994. I wanted to give women what I didn't get. And when I worked with women as they shifted out of the reproductive phase of life and into uncertain territory, I wanted to know the answers to the questions "How are you feeling?" "What are your days and nights like?" "What scares you?" "What's making you happy now?" and, most important, "Can you tell me your story? I want to hear everything."

For thirty years I have been listening hard to the stories of joy and loss, discovery and fear, freedom and disorientation from women in Transition. And for most of that time, I have been sitting at the vanguard of research at UCSF's medical school, where I've had a front-row seat to groundbreaking, impactful science. I've witnessed the emergence of real actions we can take to come into our fullness, with an increasing number of doctors and organizations focused on exactly this. I wish they were emerging faster, but the more we know, the more we ask for, the more medicine will respond with what we need.

Who Will We Be?

We are asked as children who we want to be when we grow up, and those responses are shaped by the values of the culture that we internalize, or introject. We've lived lives we wanted to live, but also the lives we thought we were supposed to manifest. For many of us it's been marriage or marriages, children or no children, careers outside or work inside the home. So much of it swept us up in a blur; so much of it is still tugging at us to fill specific roles, especially children and grandchildren. But now is the time to ask yourself, Who do you want to be today? Who do you want to be in your transition and beyond? You have decades ahead of you following the reproductive phase of life. Who do you want to be as you enter the fullness of your age? Is it a leader, an artist, a visionary, a mentor and sponsor? Is it a life filled with freedom, purpose, and focus unencumbered by the responsibilities of an earlier time? These are some of the desires I hear from women. I am obsessed with how they answer this question, and how the Transition and freedom from the fertility cycle helps us in forming a new self-image, discovering our authentic selves, and realizing our new opportunity.

I followed the science, and what I discovered is that this phase is an opportunity to grow into the wisdom and strength and resilience we've been primed for across our life span. Just as the female brain is wired for connection and communication at birth, the Upgrade allows those circuits to choose new synaptic partners that have nothing to do with the hormonal drives that dominate decision making during the reproductive phase. Changes in circuits can build a stronger and more confident sense of self, making the wisdom gained from a lifetime of experience a neurological reality.

The Transition can last between two and fourteen years. The unfolding of the Upgrade can take place in a decade and continue over the course of forty or fifty years. It's different for every woman.

From my life, the lives of the women who've come to see me, my friends, and the research, I know that freedom from the reproductive phase is an amazing, extraordinary, and now much longer period of a woman's life than ever. I think the Upgrade can even redefine what it means to be female. Here's what's possible with the Upgrade:

Directness: The massive decrease in estrogen waves changes the way the brain handles anger and disappointment. Whereas the younger female brain diverts the impulse to stand up for herself and for the values she holds dear, biologically trying to impose silence, new hormonal influences unleash those circuits. The force of the impulse to speak out will feel like driving a Maserati for the first time—it takes a little while to get used to the power. But once you do, and you see that the world didn't end, and there is no going back, nor would we want to. We shake up the status quo, redefine the rules of relationship, speak up for what's right.

Focus: The anxiety-provoking stress of multitasking is over. Multitasking and anxiety go hand in hand. We don't know which comes first, but we do know they amplify each other. With the Upgrade, we do one thing at a time. This isn't a deficit. It means you will become more engaged, more thorough, better able to concentrate. It means by being able to keep your eye on the prize, you can be more effective than you've ever been in your life; and you will no longer hesitate to tell someone who is interrupting your flow to come back later.

Validation from within: The great benefit of the cloak of invisibility of age is that we find our authenticity within. No longer driven by fertility hormones to seek external approval, we behave differently and others respond to us differently. Many find that men will listen to us not because of how we look but because of our wisdom and experience.

The return of fearlessness: In the Upgrade, the female brain is no longer stressed by its wiring being hormonally altered by 25 percent every month, and so the freedom to solidify its circuitry allows easier access to feelings of firmness and conviction unlike at any other time in a woman's life. Less concerned than ever with pleasing others, women can use this moment to build a stronger and taller platform from which to see farther and speak out.

Expansiveness: As the window gets shut tightly on the hormone storm of the Transition, the brain circuits have the opportunity to quiet. The hormonal motor that drove the hamster wheel of worry is disconnected at this time, or at least you can now identify an off-ramp. If we learn to tune out everything that interrupts the quiet—judgment, self-flagellation, loops of rumination about situations past, present, and future—a new world of options opens up. The listening circuits for hearing your own mind as well as understanding the thoughts and feelings of others can be recruited. The brain circuits for gratefulness emerge, and knowing how to optimize them determines whether you age with vitality and curiosity or become prone to depression. Compassion for self and others activates joy circuits you never knew you had, and these positive moods create the basis for robust brain health.

Freedom: The urges, obsessions, and delusions that your fertility hormones created around relationships and intimacy have released their grip. The postfertile brain is now free to explore and expand intellectually and emotionally. There is more room in your mind for contemplation, for becoming purpose oriented. Work becomes mission driven; curiosity takes center stage in decision making; a new ease takes over, even in difficult moments. While the younger female brain may pity the older woman's expanding waistline and sagging skin, we know differently. We look back with compassion toward the tortured state of mind of our younger sisters. Sighing a deep *Thank god I don't have to deal with that anymore,* we ask how we can help.

Over the decades that I worked with women at the Mood and Hormone Clinic, I've seen the power of the optimized Upgrade. By the time we've reached this age, we've been through fire. We've likely survived tragedy and begun to thrive again. We are hot molten metal, melted, molded, and burnished by life. We are the unpredictable eruption of a volcano that also builds new landmass. The Upgraded woman glows, radiates, both the sharp sword of wisdom that takes down an unjust culture and the compassion that cherishes her responsibility in creating a future for younger generations, a future she will not live to see.

The Upgrade is bold ownership, like the teen girl who knows she's got it wired and that her mom is an idiot. (Because actually, it's true in her reality.) In the Upgrade, it's the bold authority that women in the second half of life actually do have it wired; and that someday younger women and literally all men will catch up. It's knowing this, saying this, and staring down anyone who hasn't gotten with the program. It's a function of what happens when the female brain is freed from the tortuous hormonal waves that swamp and recede in daily variation during the reproductive phase.

Yes, Virginia, It's Different

When *The Female Brain* first came out, I took a lot of heat. My shocking, newsworthy premise? That female hormones and brains and male hormones and brains are not identical. That idea struck many as politically incorrect, especially other baby-boomer women like me who came of age during the women's movement. We believed that if women were ever to truly gain equality with men in society, we had to avoid emphasizing sex differences; otherwise women would lose out. Feminism itself was built upon a deep sense of inferiority received from the signals in society about who is in power and whom we answered to. And so a mandatory unisex agenda came into existence. Frankly, at the time, I bought into it as much as anyone. But then I went on to study the biology of hormones and followed the evidence—and it led me to see the clear brain differences between men and women. I suspect that future research on the hormonal impact on the brains of transgender men and women will also bolster the case.

Doing a deep dive into the evidence is how I roll, despite the push-back that evidence might prompt. And once I started digging deeper into the reams of newly emerging information about women in the second half of life, I realized there was yet another story about the female brain that I wanted to tell: the riveting, electrifying story of how things get better, things like relationships, self-care, confidence, inner strength, agency, and effectiveness. Given the messages we've received from the youth-obsessed culture about physical peaks coming so early in life, this felt counterintuitive. Because like most of us, I'd internalized what our social structures tell us through persistent pay inequity and our near invisibility in corporate leadership, politics, and research funding—that women over fifty don't matter.

For most of human history, the only way to get ahead seemed to be to agree with those in power. It's just easier to attune to the wavelength of the times. It's the compromise generations of women before us made to keep the peace, to avoid the stress of conflict. A lifetime of being seen as the side dish, the second sex, becomes part of our nervous system. Without being conscious of it, we learn to identify ourselves relative to others, female only relative to male. Taking off those blinders and stepping into our authenticity is a challenge to ourselves: to recognize that "second sex" is not who we are. We are female, as female. And we celebrate our extraordinary strengths.

Taking the Controls

For an Upgrade to happen, you need to have agency. You need to realize how much power you hold to shape the second half of your life. This is the time for creating the map for women in the postfertile, postreproductive phase of human development. The second half of a woman's life is a revelation.

If we don't think the Upgrade is possible, we won't even be able to daydream about it, recruiting the brain's powerful imaginative and planning centers to map out our own future path. We need to be inspired early to envision what we want to do in the years after forty-five. It's harder to dream when you don't have the role models or the landmarks, but if we never begin, if we never try, nothing changes.

Our mothers and grandmothers had few role models for dreaming into what it means to be female in and of itself. Today we have more women to help guide us. And if we make the most of the opportunity, future generations will be able to go even further than we will. Change is possible. Think about how much the world has shifted for the LGBTQ+ community in our lifetimes. Women are 51 percent of the world's population. We can make the Upgrade available for them.

How do we make the world a place that holds hope for older women? As wages for jobs mostly held by women, like waitressing, childcare, cleaning, and healthcare—both in the home and professionally—decline, many will be left without savings or a retirement plan. How many will die early because of lack of access to medical care? Women in the second half of life will take the brunt of the impact of the wealth gap, especially BIPOC women. And the world remains silent as it happens, focusing instead on the loss of jobs for white males.

For the most part, what we have been expected to do in the second half of life is to continue the caretaking role: of older husbands, grandchildren, extremely aged parents and in-laws. Men don't even think about taking on the responsibility of caring for a family member as long as there is a woman around to do it. After decades of raising children, doing the majority of the housework, holding down the second shift at home even if we are the primary breadwinner, again we become unpaid caretakers; our emotional and financial resources are drained, making it impossible to work, to be productive, to soar.

But for anyone who thinks women in the Upgrade are takers, data is proving we are makers. Women over fifty start new businesses at a higher rate than any other group, offering opportunity to others, becoming the nation's economic and caretaking shoulders. To be seen, you must see yourself. And at this moment, when we have survived so many crises both personal and societal, we have the wisdom, stability, courage, and self-knowledge to trust ourselves to make it through. We need to change the conversation in the culture, but more important is the conversation inside our own heads.

———

The world has been in warrior mode for too long, ensnared in one constant zero-sum battle fueled by a testosterone-driven addiction to risk, on the trading floor and on the world stage. Warrior mode, driven by a personality trait of dominance that is specifically male, is not how society progresses. It is not how culture survives. It's time to balance humanity with a different brain style, one that holds as its core value community and preservation of life. The Upgraded female brain has the ability to balance human culture.

My purpose in writing this book is to give you validation for having good ideas, for having a great life, for having a life of your own that you build and choose. And to encourage you to endorse one another as women and endorse ourselves as a result. Amplification has to be put into practice by each and every one of us, each and every day.

In the Upgrade, neurobiology is there to support us in shedding the skin of the fertile-phase identity and in embracing and stepping purposefully into a more authentic, powerful version of ourselves. Ask yourself now, What is your idea of freedom? If money and physical vulnerability were taken out of the equation, what would you do? Who would you be? In the Upgrade, we can begin to dream as if everything were possible. I am here to help you dream.

The Crux of Being Female

Chapter 2

Biological systems love balance. They yearn for, they crave, an easy collaboration, signals communicating like clockwork, pinging gentle reminders to keep everything in working order. They fight for equilibrium. In a biological organism, this drive toward the status quo, otherwise known as health, is called homeostasis. The process turns genes on and off like a massive, multidimensional Rube Goldberg system responding with tiny, rapid countermeasures to any disturbance, from the molecular to a giant external force. Proteins and molecules are generated that help establish balance or demand an action that will right the ship—eat, sleep, snuggle, run—ensuring a smooth operating system that supports health and strength. The pendulum swings perpetually, never finding the perfect middle. This fight to keep things calm and the same is a basic principle for all living things.

So imagine a biological system in which the default drive for balance is buffeted daily by a wild chemical storm, bringing waves of neurohormones determined to evoke an action, a response, a new behavior from the system. As estrogen, progesterone, testosterone, DHEA, cortisol, and many others shift in hourly, daily, weekly, monthly waves, it isn't just menses that is affected and thrown off balance: The brain, the body's entire nervous system, is alternately provoked and soothed, each hormonal molecule demanding an action to further the survival of the system itself. The female brain is pushed by strong hormonal waves to mate, to flirt, to curl up by a fire, to eat chocolate cake, to rage, to hug, to rightly scold, to speak an unvarnished truth no one is ready to hear.

Waves are one of the most powerful and efficient physical forces in existence. Whether ripples in a pond or a twenty-foot storm surge, waves change everything they touch, battering boulders into pebbles, pulverizing shells into sand. Their push builds a coastline, depositing landmass, broken glass, shells, seaweed, ships, sometimes living creatures. Their pull is equally strong, the undertow dragging away what the tide has tossed up, gutting coastlines, digging a steep drop to the ocean floor in deep blue waters.

The Keys are a small chain of islands off the Florida peninsula extending southwest on the limestone, sandy soil, and coral reef upon which most of the state rests. On the west side of the Keys, facing the Florida Bay and the Gulf of Mexico, is calm, perfectly clear cerulean water, sandbars that extend for miles, through which residents wade barefoot all day in the warm, knee-deep sea. The smooth, sandy bottom, marked by soft wave patterns, is clearly visible. The shoreline is regular, inhabited by small creatures at home in shallow saltwater. Dotted with white coral boulders, the gentle tide doesn't wash up much seaweed, nor does it erode the shallows noticeably unless it is hit by an unusually large storm.

The landmass of the islands is narrow, in places less than two miles across. Around the middle of the chain, a ten-minute walk east delivers you to the Atlantic side. There, the ocean is rough, the water murky. Though it is made of the same sand, limestone, warm saltwater, and coral rock, it looks nothing like the western shore. Seaweed carpets the rocky beach like the world's thickest shag. Sea urchins and stingrays hover near the water's edge, hidden in the underwater growth; the shallows are littered with rocks that slice through the most calloused feet. Eroded by the constant pull of a strong undertow, the shore drops off quickly to depths more accommodating to larger, predatory sea life. This is the shore upon which you will find sea glass, its jagged edges rounded, surface softened and turned opaque by the abrasive tides and sand.

Though the elements are the same, the shoreline carved by waves has undergone undeniable structural change. A rock on the calmer gulf side has a structure different from one battered by the relentless push and pull of the open Atlantic Ocean. Dump a truckload of sand on the western shore and it will establish a small beach. Do the same on the Atlantic side and it will be sucked out to sea within a few days.

Waves of Hormones

Waves impact human beings in the form of cycles of behavior-driving hormones. Cortisol, a hormone released by the adrenal glands, flows in a wave that during its push phase wakes us up, keeps our memory sharp, helps us feel alert and eager to learn. At its height in the morning, we feel faster on our feet and excited for the day. During the pull phase, when cortisol bottoms out at 3:00 or 4:00 P.M., we yearn for a nap, chocolate, a caffeinated soda, coffee, anything to recover the day's earlier freshness. If we ride the pull of the cortisol wave out, we relax, slow down, become tired, and if all goes well, another wave of hormones helps us sleep soundly through the night, giving the brain a chance to be cleared of toxins and overgrowth accrued from the stimuli of the day. If anything interrupts this wave—staying up too late, crossing time zones, having a big fight with a loved one, or a deeply traumatic experience—the brain's neurocircuitry is rewired as the cortisol wave becomes irregular, setting off other waves that also behave unpredictably. We might spend half the night awake in agitated, worried rumination. In the case of trauma, if the adrenal hormones get stuck in the *on* position, the brain's circuitry changes so dramatically that it becomes impossible to learn, to relax, or to perceive circumstances and people as anything but threatening.

All terrain, including the neurocircuitry that drives thoughts, emotion, and behavior, is altered by waves. The diurnal cortisol wave is common to both female and male. As long as we stay on a fairly regular schedule of waking, exercising, eating, and sleeping, and we are not facing biological disruption, the waves are less dramatic, and the terrain is less dramatically impacted.

Over the course of a lifetime, the male brain and nervous system will experience the waves common to all human beings, daily ups and downs of chemicals that drive waking, sleeping, circulation, breathing, hunger, thirst, thinking, learning, sex, and emotion. In the male brain at puberty, the pituitary pings the testicles to produce testosterone, and the sex drive ignites in earnest. For boys this feels emotionally dramatic as the urgency of physical intimacy becomes a dominant drive, but the testosterone wave itself is anything but. Testosterone rises and falls daily in a duet with the cortisol wave, making morning erections the strongest. But the male brain's lifelong melody is a single and uncomplicated wave, rising to an early-adult crescendo and falling at a gentle slope into old age. The testosterone wave runs predictably atop the reliable counterpoint of daily hormonal waves controlling other basic drives.

But something different is brewing in the female brain. Between six and thirteen years old, a girl's hypothalamus pings the pituitary to activate several hormonal waves. One is the adrenal wave, which wakes up the little hormone control centers, the adrenal glands, that sit on top of the kidneys, asking for a wave of the androgen DHEA. DHEA, a little bundle of energy, excitement, and zest for life, is often called the mother hormone, because it converts into both estrogen and testosterone. Testosterone, in females as well as males, drives interest in sex.

The tween girl's behavior becomes a bit testy. "Don't touch my hair." "Stop looking at me." "Don't talk to me." "Leave me alone." Other effects of the adrenal wave are the arousal of her nervous system through cortisol, adrenaline, and DHEA, which in the right amounts optimize her ability to both learn new things and remember them and kicks up the vigilance essential to detecting danger and acting successfully in the face of it. It's adrenaline and a bit of cortisol that will put her on alert about going out late at night alone, or heighten her awareness when at some point in her life she walks unaccompanied through a large, deserted parking garage.

This same process of the hypothalamus pinging the pituitary sets off another hormonal interaction, a unique and complex dance of waves crashing and receding on the shores of the brain and the ovaries. Two chemicals from the pituitary, luteinizing hormone (LH) and follicle-stimulating hormone (FSH), will send the ovaries the signal to make the estrogen needed to prepare eggs to be ripened for fertilization and to line the uterus with a soft cushion for a fertilized egg to attach to. For most women, there will be an eightfold increase in estrogen during their cycle. Estrogen pulls behind it a little wagon of oxytocin, the bonding hormone, a strong neurochemical pairing for females. The more estrogen, the more oxytocin. Though males also have oxytocin, the levels are much lower. On the push side of the wave, estrogen and oxytocin help drive flirtatious and warm, cuddly behavior in females.

These waves of LH, FSH, estrogen, oxytocin, and testosterone temporarily reorganize brain networks and stimulate qualities like memory, language, and affection, peaking around ovulation. A few days after ovulation, estrogen crashes, leaving mostly progesterone and a testosterone cattle prod of edginess. The pituitary withdraws the wave of LH and FSH as the ovaries produce the undertow of progesterone that after four days drags away the extroverted, outgoing bubbliness, pulling with it, like strands of seaweed lost in the tide, the brain circuits for interest in social connection and the crisp ability to communicate. While progesterone sends signals to the uterine lining to keep building, it also drives the urge to turn inward, lowers mental acuity, and increases pain sensitivity. For most women, it's an eightfold increase in progesterone at this time. Progesterone, in the form of its metabolite, allopregnanolone (ALLO), dials up the brain's GABAergic activity. GABA is the brain's natural Valium; it is the major calming system in the brain. The system-wide GABAergic activity is what puts the brakes on the growth, connectivity, and stimulation pushed by estrogen. If we didn't have those brakes, we'd be having seizures all the time, or at least be edgy and anxious. The entire nervous system has GABAergic receptors that are influenced by the metabolite of progesterone, ALLO. It sends a calming, antianxiety signal, and is what creates that comfy, cozy time of the month when you mostly want to stay home, watch romantic movies, and eat cake or ice cream. ALLO is what makes you feel incredibly sedated during the first half of pregnancy. But all good things must come to an end, and you know what's next: PMS, bloating, cramps, and blood that will come with the dramatic drop in progesterone, which pulls ALLO down with it. In the last two days of the cycle, when progesterone bottoms out, preparing the uterine lining to shed, our edgy down mood colors everything. We cry during commercials showing adults hugging babies and puppies. An upset over a personal issue can signal the brain to make it feel like the beginning of a global catastrophe.

Negative and Positive

The human brain is notoriously skewed by negativity bias, making it easy to laser-focus in on one little bad thing that happened, while shutting out all the good. When we lived in the wild, this particular cognitive bias helped burn into our memory the location of the watering hole where we saw a lion eating an antelope, so that we would warn others away. Now negativity bias is what makes us hungry for scary alerts or updated news of a disaster, and it explains why good news dissipates quickly. Some neuroscientists describe this as the brain having Velcro for negativity and Teflon for positivity.

Amplified by the steep drop-off of progesterone—around an eightfold decrease—every month, the female brain circuits can get dragged out to a depressive sea. If progesterone is chemically consumed via birth control pill use or given in too high a dose in hormone therapy (HT), it can dramatically increase depression in a susceptible woman and double her risk for suicide.

As waves of neurochemicals crash and subside in a woman's body, they flip on and off genetic switches and receptors that alter connections in the female brain up to 25 percent every twenty-six to thirty-five or so days. The waves drive radical reality differences week to week—from feeling friendly, smart, and positive to having a mental filter that interprets comments and interactions with others as negative and critical. The pull and tug of these waves has a high-frequency amplitude; over the course of a woman's life, this dramatic churn remakes the female brain's terrain somewhere around five hundred times.

Pregnancy, childbirth, and child-rearing bring a strong, steady wind, inalterably high tides, climate change, and the formation of new landmass, all of which make the female brain think, act, and live for the two, three, four, ten, or however many children she has. Presaged by fogginess during pregnancy, the "self" hard drive in the brain is wiped for recoding to put offspring ahead of all. The lack of mental clarity is a side effect of the major brain resets that happen during puberty, pregnancy, postpartum, Transition, and Upgrade. The wrong words come out, we can't find the keys or remember to calendar the meeting we just arranged—all evidence of the frontal cortex shutting down in order to allow the limbic emotional brain to take over the rewiring that undeniably and irrevocably alters the female biological landscape.

For every action there is an equal and opposite reaction. As the pendulum of the homeostatic process swings hard in the opposite direction of a change, the action will overshoot its mark in its attempt to land in a precise and static equipoise that—in an ever-shifting environment—can never come. In the female brain, the course corrections come rapid fire, every day for a duration of around thirty-five years.

The Transition into the Upgrade can make an already wild fight for homeostasis even more dramatic.

Sometime in a woman's late thirties to early forties, production of adrenal DHEA (which, remember, converts into both estrogen and testosterone) and ovarian estrogen begin to slightly decrease. The hypothalamus and pituitary gland, estrogen junkies since puberty, will send a strong spurt of LH and FSH, demanding relief from withdrawal symptoms. The ovaries comply by spiking a tsunami of estrogen, knocking the brain and body even further off balance. Estrogen has a profound impact on cognition, memory, mental acuity, and mood, and a spike in estrogen can bring about scattered thinking and a crazy amount of testiness. The estrogen spike is followed by a dramatic undertow of progesterone. The outgoing affection caused by estrogen and oxytocin gets interrupted by irritability, sadness, scattered thinking, and pessimism, especially when progesterone drops harder after a more precipitous rise. The woman in transition becomes testy. The behavior provoked by erratic waves of hormones can range from "Don't touch me" to "Get out of my life."

Cycles become irregular when lack of ovulation leads to no estrogen or progesterone surge; it's ovulation that signals for the continuing buildup of the uterine lining. Usually progesterone enters as estrogen declines, keeping the lining plump and in place. If there is no pregnancy, progesterone abruptly declines, signaling the lining to shed. Without progesterone, ALLO doesn't show up to calm the brain and nervous system. And without progesterone's decline, the uterine lining won't shed until it becomes too heavy. At that point, bleeding can become profuse.

Not every woman will experience the shift in the same way, but for the 30 percent who go through a dramatic version of the Transition, the wild push-pull of this neurochemical storm lasts between two and fourteen years, the pituitary's demand for hormones driving extreme swings of mood and behavior. The pulsing GnRH (gonadotropin-releasing hormone) cells in the hypothalamus, which started the whole process in puberty, spike their signals until they get stuck on high, like Maria Callas straining the top of her range, screeching out an endless note to an empty and darkened concert hall.

The biology of the body is tied up in survival. Anytime a system begins shutting down, it creates panic in the organism. That panic, transmitted via the nervous system, becomes an unconscious driver of thought, emotion, and behavior. And does it have an outlet? Can it find relief? The prefrontal cortex, the quintessential human brain area that generates insight, can calm the panicked amygdala and tell us through analysis that this is not life-threatening. We can learn to understand the difference between biological panic and a genuine threat; that the version of us that's projected by neurohormones is not the true us, even though it doesn't feel that way when the waves are crashing in the storm.

There is no male corollary to this process. Though the basic brain material of female and male is mostly the same, waves create measurable structural difference. Just like the two shores of the Florida Keys or the Caribbean and Pacific coasts of Costa Rica, environment, structure, and experience are radically altered by the force and frequency of waves.

Resilience

Waves are the crux of being female, burnishing the essential female power of resilience. Resilience is the ability to quickly return to a zone of well-being when the system, or the person, has been knocked out of phase. Resilience is the single strongest factor that contributes not only to the survival of a system but to the possibility that it will reach its full, maximized potential. Resilience can be built and enhanced only by the buffeting of destabilizing forces, like the waves experienced by the female brain.

The ability to surf those waves in the midst of neurochemical storms is reflected in female psychology as the core of our courage, our strength, our will, our agency, our power. The waves cause just enough suffering to help us connect with our best qualities. The dance of youth, of hormones that trapped us in the arena of nonstop acquisition—marriage, children, career, money—ends when the ovaries go deaf to the brain's demanding signal for estrogen, testosterone, and progesterone.

The crashing of those dramatic waves is wiping the hard drive to prepare it for the Upgrade, a state that can quiet the brain's hypervigilance around survival, kids, and relationships and remove the filters of worry over how we appear to others. When you pass through the door to the Upgrade, your ability to see your most positive and authentic self is no longer clouded. You've walked through fire to come into your true power. You've emerged from the storm into wisdom. What you thought were feminine powers, the minor female powers of sexuality, you realize were just decoration.

Community

As the minds and nervous systems of war veterans are changed and as they are bonded by their experience, so it goes with females. Communities of veterans come together with a shared sense of one another. Women in the Transition and the Upgrade know instinctively that someone who wasn't on the front lines of this particular hormonal battle will never completely understand us.

We are not, in the Upgrade, an old version of ourselves returned. The girl we left behind remains in the past. We have been changed forever by decades lived in a biological war zone, pushed edge to edge every week, chemicals flipping genes connected to fighting disease, stress, sex drive, and mental acuity on and off at a breakneck pace. That war zone has made us who we are, visceral beings, using the complete self to sense and understand people and reality.

In the Upgrade we recognize that our visceral sense makes us stronger. It adds to our intuition, the absorption of information that happens so quickly there is little time to unpack what's coming in. It pushes to the forefront our more available mirror neurons, which allow us to sense another's nervous system, to vibrate with understanding of others. It's not that men don't have similar visceral systems; it's that they don't have the hormonal waves that have sensitized and cracked them open for fully optimized availability.

Unless a Y chromosome comes along, every single embryo will be female. A uterus, ovaries, and clitoris will develop in the absence of a steady production of testosterone. Female is the primordial gender. Waves are nature's primordial force. Male is the female rib, the second sex, unburnished by waves, functioning in a narrower zone of well-being. Female power dances outside that zone, knowing that shaking up normalcy will end in transformation, not destruction.

Out of the wildness that goes with our biology comes an innate ferociousness. Characteristically female, it pushes us to call things out when they go awry, to scream for change when the larger system is in danger, to demand safer conditions when our sisters are burned alive in a shirtwaist factory, to withstand ridicule as we fight to save the planet from disastrous, man-made, *man*-made climate change. That is who we are; this is a great thing, not something to be covered over or stifled or ignored. Our biological extremes are what can make a difference emotionally and socially. We are the change agent. We become capacious in being able to hold so much energy and potential.

Think what happens when the push and pull of all that change settles, how much more resilient and prepared we are for daily life changes, what an opportunity it is for creativity to come to the fore as brain circuits that were engaged nearly full time in managing the waves are now free to be deployed as we see fit, creating a new reality for what could be the best time of our lives. Biology is destiny, unless you know what it's doing to you. The question is, into which destiny would you like to emerge?

Transitioning into the Upgrade

Chapter 3

My patient Carole is an in-house lawyer with a regional bank in Dallas. At forty-seven, she's been married to Ron for twenty-two years. They have one daughter, and Ron is clearly devoted to both of the women in his life. But lately there seems to have been a lot of stress in their relationship. Carole feels criticized all the time. It's resulting in lots of fights; their old ability to communicate and solve problems seems to have evaporated. Ron feels bewildered as Carole rebuffs his affection one minute and apologizes for being distant the next. "I just want to be able to make her happy again," he tells me when we meet, "but I don't seem to be able to do that right now."

For the first time, things have also been rough at work. Carole has had a meteoric and charmed career, and for years everything she touched turned to gold. Lately, it feels like her hot streak has gone cold. Nothing seems to go right and her boss has become relentlessly impatient. She's been misreading situations and sending flame-o-gram emails for which she finds herself apologizing a day later. She's never been the most laid-back person, but her temper is now hair-trigger, and she's struggling to keep a lid on it.

And then the unthinkable happens: Her boss tells her in their weekly meeting that her contract won't be renewed. She has never lost a job in her entire life, and she is faced with forty-eight hours to pack up a twenty-five-year-career. Where she had always been high energy, ebullient, and optimistic, now Ron holds her every night while she sobs herself to sleep. It's like the bottom dropped out of some innate toughness she had always relied upon in difficult circumstances. It seems like it happened all of a sudden, but, ageism of corporations aside, the hormonal roller coaster caused by the process of wiping her brain's hard drive and getting it ready to be rewired for the Upgrade has been pushing her to this precipice for a few years now. She's had fallings-out with a number of old friends and colleagues over perceived slights. By the time she came to see me, she had partially blown up her life.

Although Carole's situation is complicated and may seem extreme, there were strong biological reasons for what was happening. The physical and identity transition that takes place at this stage in a woman's brain is profound. I want to acknowledge and validate that for you. In this moment when you may feel less like yourself than ever, when your old tricks for calming down, sleeping it off, or losing weight stop working, it's not just stress, and it's not made up. It's real, it's physical, and it's in your brain. You can't just Zen out and think, *Let it go,* as some of Carole's friends suggested, and hope that the symptoms will magically disappear. You can't command your body like you used to, with healthy eating, exercise, and habits, to just figure it out and expect to return to your old normal. While good habits help us turn the Transition into an Upgrade, they won't prevent the symptoms of the Transition for many of us.

What the body is trying to figure out is not that simple. After decades of predictable cycles, suddenly everything just feels off. Cycles may be shorter or longer. You may be bleeding less or more. This isn't just about volume and the calendar: They are hormonal events that can shift dramatically how we feel about ourselves, our lives, our relationships, our careers. And what you are going through or have gone through already may mean you have to get used to being a new and different person, growing into a new and different body, having a new and different sense of who you are. Carole and I were able to find a way forward that worked for her. It's not the same solution for everyone. In this case, hormone therapy (HT) solved a lot. "It wasn't that I became my old self," she told me when I asked her about how she was feeling. "It's that it helped me emerge into who I was becoming without feeling like I was alternately being dragged away from the shore and tossed back onto the beach. A new job is next!"

For women, there are estrogen and progesterone receptors on every single organ, not just the brain. Not surprisingly, as production of the hormones declines, the impact can feel profound. For many, this time is a fundamental transformation of our physical and emotional identity, almost like a reincarnation taking place within a single lifetime. By going through my own Transition, and by holding the space for so many women as they have gone through it, I have come to respect the process deeply.

As you read this chapter, at some point you are going to think, *Dr. Louann, you've sold me a bill of goods. This book should be called* The Downgrade. And I hear you. Like anything in life, good comes with bad. There are some rough spots during the transition physically, emotionally, and in terms of finding help. None of them are your fault; and the most important message is to learn to become your own advocate. I want to send you in to your doctor armed with the right questions and the best information, so that you can recruit her to your team. Make sure to fill that team with the most supportive and knowledgeable friends and family. If you haven't Transitioned, talk to a friend who has already Upgraded about coming to appointments with you. She might ask questions you may not think of. It's an uncertain time of life; it's so reassuring to have a village in your corner to help you figure out how to make this stage the most productive and rewarding.

Ladies! Start Your Spreadsheets!

It wasn't that long ago, in the nineteenth century, when all it took was a single act of rage, a missed menstrual cycle, or an extended period of grief over the loss of a family member to have a woman sent away. Though we can express ourselves now without being locked in an asylum, the echo of repression is still apparent in how alone and isolated most of us feel during one of the most extraordinary transformations any human being will endure. If you've already gone through the Transition, I hope this map will give you some clarity about the territory through which you've traveled. If you haven't, while it is different for everyone, here are some landmarks you can look out for. If you're still having periods and you're not using your calendar, a spreadsheet, or an app to track your cycles, now is the time to start.

During the Transition, just as in puberty, hormones can cause wild emotional swings. That process alone can cause feelings of isolation, as we wonder if what we are going through is normal, if anyone else has ever had our experience, if we are going crazy or not. If you went through the Transition early, you didn't have your peers to talk to. If you went through it late, your friends who had already completed it might not have wanted to talk about it either. "I asked my friend Ceci," Carole said, "who is about twenty years older than I am, about it. All she had to say was that she remembered being very concerned about her health at that time. But that was it. No details other than she threw some jewelry into the Hudson River when she got mad at her ex-husband." Carole laughed at the memory.

Let's start with a look backward, so that you can orient yourself. Unless you're on hormonal birth control or the pill during the years before the Transition, the pituitary sends out two hormones, luteinizing hormone (LH) and follicle-stimulating hormone (FSH), like clockwork to regulate your cycles. These signals, which are of course blocked by the pill, request that two jobs get done. One prompts the maturation of an estrogen-producing egg follicle, and the other gets the follicle to launch the egg through the fallopian tube to the uterus (ovulation). The estrogen from the follicle nudges the uterus to build a cushy lining in case that egg is fertilized and needs to implant. Whenever estrogen goes up, up with it goes oxytocin, the hormone that triggers an affectionate, cuddly, trusting, connecting state of mind and behavior. After ovulation, that same ovarian follicle turns into an entirely different endocrine organ and produces comfy, cozy, stay-at-home-and-take-care-of-yourself progesterone to keep the thickening uterine lining in place. If the egg isn't fertilized, no implantation happens and progesterone plummets. It is dramatic; we can get pretty cranky as ALLO drops like a rock, and the cushy lining bleeds off.

We are born with about a million eggs, our lifetime supply. By the time we are teenagers, the ovaries' supply of eggs is about half a million. Every month, nine or ten follicles race to maturity. The best, most viable gets picked for ovulation. By our late thirties, the supply is anywhere between ten thousand and fifteen thousand and exponentially declining. Over many decades, as with all aging cells, the DNA of the eggs degrades and we have fewer viable eggs. Genetic mutations in an egg often mean it won't mature or, if it does, those mutations become fatal to an embryo; in less than ten weeks or so, the body's system, sensing that the embryo isn't viable, finds a way to end such a pregnancy via miscarriage. As we run out of mutation-free eggs, none mature. No maturing eggs means no follicular estrogen, which means much less oxytocin and no progesterone. Without those potent neurochemicals signaling the brain the way it's used to being signaled, we already feel a bit destabilized.

You Are Here ⬇⬇

Looking backward, we can see that there are four stages to the Transition. The first, the Pre-Transition, begins on average at around thirty-seven. It happens as the number of viable eggs declines and fewer follicles are formed, impacting the amount of sex hormones produced each month. You might notice a bit more anxiety just before your period, a bit more trouble cooling off after an intense aerobic workout, or a little bit of heat or sweating at night. Your sleep might be interrupted by this around the time of your period.

The Early Transition, around forty to forty-five, is marked by more noticeable sleep disruption—you may find yourself fully drenched or wake up with the covers thrown off—at least once a week or so. In the Early Transition you might experience occasional irregular bleeding: less volume and fewer days, a bit more blood over a day or two more, skipped bleeding, or midmonth bleeding. This happens because of an increase in a common, normal event: anovulation, or an eggless cycle.

During the fertility phase, we might have one such anovulatory cycle per year, in which there is no viable egg and so the ovary doesn't form an ovulatory follicle. Remember that the follicle becomes its own mini endocrine organ, stimulating the production and withdrawal of hormones that can shift our brain's cognition and mood throughout the month. As we get closer to the Upgrade, we have more such cycles. The sign of anovulation is that your cycle is shorter than usual, maybe by as little as one to three days. If you have two or three short cycles in a year, going from, say, twenty-eight down to twenty-seven or twenty-six or twenty-five days, this can be a sign of the Mid-Transition, and it can happen years before you ever miss a period.

We have all been taught to look for hot flashes and mood swings as the first sign of the Transition, but trust me, it's easy to deny they are happening. It's easy to blame your car's climate control, the air conditioner or bedding in your home, stress, or a tough emotional situation for the first few months or even years of the Transition. But this quantitative marker—the shortening of cycles—is a more reliable sign than testing hormone levels and less subjective than sweating or irritability, though by the Mid- and Late Transition, you may be experiencing sleep interruption on a nightly basis. At the same time, if you're not paying attention, the sign is easy to miss, like crossing a state line at seventy-five miles per hour and whizzing right past a sun-bleached marker. If you haven't tracked your period, now is the time, that is, if you aren't on the pill. Your calendar will tell you everything you need to know about what's coming. If you're on the pill, the only way to find out what's happening with your cycles is to stop taking it.

If you're experiencing between three and ten shortened cycles per year, then welcome to the Late Transition, the gateway to the Upgrade. The average age at the end of this stage is fifty-one, but it's not the same for everyone. The better indicator is a measurable biological event. And for many women, the neurohormonal impact of this time can be profound.

When there's no ripened egg, the very precise hormonal choreography of pituitary, ovaries, and uterus, of LH, estrogen, FSH, and progesterone, becomes a bit loose—like going from the lockstep of the *Swan Lake* corps de ballet to modern improvisation. When there is no maturing egg follicle, the brain doesn't get the estrogen it's used to. So in its demand for more, a strong FSH spike from the brain's pituitary forces a big follicular estrogen spike and an ovulation. Without ovulation, however, there is no progesterone surge, thus no sudden drop that gets the uterine lining to bleed off. Instead, the lining keeps thickening. When it becomes too heavy to hold in place, the law of gravity takes over; the sheer weight and volume of tissue and blood can cause it to shed even without the progesterone trigger.

The amount of blood can be frightening, and a lot of women will think they are miscarrying or dying. Clots the size of golf balls may plop into the toilet. Your bed might look like a crime scene. One friend said it sounded like she was peeing when she took out her tampon over the toilet. If the brain isn't sensing enough estrogen, it can also blast out an FSH spike midcycle, spurring the growth of an entirely new set of follicles before the body has time to deal with the first set. Like trains getting backed up in a station, these LOOP (luteal out-of-phase) or stacked cycles can lead to prolonged bleeding as the uterine lining gets out-of-whack signals and keeps building. The time between cycles continues to shorten, until some women feel like their cycles have flipped—they might bleed for twenty-one days and stop for five. This is not uncommon in the Mid- and Late Transition.

"The best advice I got was to carry a much larger purse," Carole said of her bouts with heavy bleeding. "I had to pack whole boxes of tampons and pads. I needed clean undies and a plastic bag for any that got soaked. A friend told me to give away my white pants, because by the time I would stop bleeding long enough to wear them, they would either be too small or out of style.

"The worst," Carole continued, "was being at a dinner party and feeling a leak about to spring. First, there's the fear of ruining your friend's upholstery. Then the worry of what will happen when you finally stand up. Worse still is that clear white plastic powder room garbage can with no lining. They became my mortal enemy! I started carrying a roll of small opaque garbage bags along with my other supplies."

As many as 25 percent of women will have what we call flooding. Yes, that is the term for it. And no, this isn't due to stress, though travel across time zones and hemispheres might intensify it. At any age, when we do something to throw off the body's circadian rhythm—the wake/sleep/eat hormone cycles—it can destabilize all other hormone signals, including those for ovulation and menstruation. "I used to practice the rhythm method, since I was so regular and was really good at predicting my own fertility," said Liz, fifty-four. "But during my medical internship in my late twenties, I was on call and up all night every fourth night. I couldn't figure out my cycles to save my life during that time, and I had a couple of oopsies with my boyfriend."

"Frequency of overseas travel was one question my ob-gyn asked me when I came in concerned about heavy bleeding," said Patricia, forty-nine, a new patient of mine. Her OB had been in practice for more than forty years and had seen everything. He noticed that the women he treated in their forties and fifties who had busy travel schedules often complained of heavy bleeding. "Over the course of three weeks around the holidays, I went from winter in New York to summer solstice in Brazil, then winter solstice in Norway. By the third week of January, I was inca-pacitated." An actress with a touring company, Patricia continued, "I started to pack an extra suitcase and plastic bags for damp clothes that I had washed but didn't have a chance to dry. I never go anywhere now without hydrogen peroxide and Q-tips. It's the best for cleaning blood out of clothes, chairs, couches, sheets, whatever."

I want to reassure you that while much of this is normal, everyone approaches coping with symptoms differently. Some women feel fine riding out the waves until they subside, confident in the body to take its time, even if that happens over the course of years. Others want to beat the body into submission. But the vast majority can find relief in a combination of approaches: medication that may include HT or an antidepressant, or perhaps an outpatient procedure to reduce the heft of the uterine lining.

One caution: Heavy bleeding can sometimes be a sign of uterine cancer. Since 91 percent of those with uterine cancer have had heavy bleeding, it's a good precaution to get a biopsy of your uterine tissue if your doctor recommends it; but chances are, heavy bleeding just means you're in the early stages of the Transition. Also, if you are bleeding a lot, get your hemoglobin and hematocrit levels checked for anemia. It's possible you will need an iron supplement to get you through this time. If you've suffered from anemia because of heavy bleeding, have your doctor perform an RDW test, which measures red blood cell width, even after you've completed the Transition. That will tell you if your bone marrow, which produces your red blood cells, has caught up in production. Some women need to stay on an iron supplement after the Transition until the Upgrade is complete.

"The hardest part for me," Patricia continued, "was that my old strategies for dealing with cycles started having the opposite effect. Exercise had always helped with cramps and with moodiness. I used to do back-to-back Zumba and cardio-burn classes at the gym on Saturday mornings before heading off to see friends. But once I hit the Transition, those classes would knock me out for two or three hours. And oh, baby, I couldn't believe the cramps."

Exercise can sometimes make Transition cramps worse, especially if you have fibroids. The uterus, which is made of smooth muscle—the type of muscle over which we have no conscious control—also has special little spiral arteries that feed blood to it. If those muscles and arteries didn't contract during menstruation, we would bleed to death. That process of spasm is what makes us feel the pain of cramps and is intensified during exercise. If you think you knew what bad cramps felt like, honey, those of the Transition can be of a whole new order.

"I remember doing a session with a trainer one morning," said Patricia, "and later that night I was curled in a ball on the couch in tears from the pain. Advil helped a little, but not much. After a lifetime of exercise and activity, my doctors were telling me to sleep, rest, stay quiet, and relax. That was really hard advice to take, but ultimately it worked."

The chemicals of the prostaglandin system can make things contract or relax throughout the body. The prostaglandin system is what causes those smooth muscles and spiral arteries to contract and cut off the blood supply to the uterine lining. Progesterone withdrawal, just prior to monthly bleeding, triggers hyperreactivity of the prostaglandin system, intensifying the spasm of pain. Cramps are obviously not evolutionarily adaptive—anything that puts us flat on our backs is a bad idea living in the wild. But Mother Nature thought it's better to have cramps than to bleed to death. During the Transition, when hormones start to go off balance, pain sensitivity is also heightened.

The only thing that helps is to stay ahead of the pain. By the time you have full-blown cramps, it's too late for Advil, Motrin, or any other medicines that impact the prostaglandin system to have a big impact. This means tuning in to those first twinges and popping the right NSAID (not aspirin since it causes more bleeding) in order to inhibit the muscle spasm that causes cramping. "That was one of the single most helpful things you told me," said Patricia during a session. "If I was bleeding, I learned to take Advil before exercising, and it worked to keep the cramps in check. It meant I could be a bit more active again."

Et Tu, Estrogen?

Estrogen has for most of your life been your best friend, your driver of language facility, of social connection, sex, and affection. Estrogen is the great preserver of memory in the brain, the great protector of mood and of cognitive functioning in women. Some doctors call it nature's Prozac. But during the Transition, too much of a good thing can create some hairy situations both physically and emotionally.

In addition to building up the uterine lining, estrogen makes fibroids grow like crazy. Most women develop small ones in their thirties, but during the Transition they can become grapefruit-sized or larger, and women of African descent have an increased risk of developing them. During my transition at fifty-three, I had giant fibroids pushing on my bladder that made me pee as often as during the third trimester of pregnancy. Forget about sex. On most days there was a "Don't come near me" sign hanging from my pelvis. Between the cramps, heavier bleeding, and discomfort from fibroids pressing against other organs, the shop was closed.

That's the physical part. Now for the emotions.

Estrogen stimulates growth of brain synapses, intensifies their connections, and reorganizes brain networks. That's why during the early part of normal cycles, we are talkative, we are more outgoing, and our brains feel like they are on high-octane fuel. Growth is great as long as there is a careful gardener, stimulated by progesterone, eventually coming along to cut the weeds, clip the hedges, trim the trees, and clean up the trash. But if the body gets into progesterone deficit, as it does for many women during this time, there is no gardener to do her job in the brain or the uterus. Overgrowth in both areas can result. In the brain, sleep is the best opportunity for neural pruning and taking out the trash; but sleep can be a challenge during the Transition, and without enough of it, focusing and trying to find emotional stability can become a major struggle.

In the Late Transition, the sputtering hormones can trigger mood drops and sadness as the brain tries to adjust to the changes in its neurochemical reality. This is a moment when you may need extra support for dealing with fear or sadness, especially if your Transition is longer than about five years or you've had a major life upheaval.

As cycles continue to shorten, erratic dips in estrogen and progesterone from the ovaries cause neurocircuit withdrawal, setting off alarm bells in the brain. Many doctors recommend testing FSH levels to determine whether or not you've entered the Transition. But in my experience, this test is unreliable until you are already done with the Transition. During this phase, the level can be wildly erratic. It can change by the hour, depending upon whether or not there is an estrogen spike from a follicle that's been forced to squeeze more out. Higher estrogen lowers FSH. If you happen to get tested during an estrogen spike, your FSH will look normal or low, and your doctor will tell you that you are not in the Transition, even though you might be.

Think about what a test result like this might do to your sense of reality if you have been living with wild mood swings, erratic cycles, warm flushes, and just not feeling like yourself anymore. You walk into your doctor's office, hoping for some answers. You get your FSH level tested and it comes back normal. Think about the cognitive dissonance of having to figure out which source is more reliable: your own experience or the data from the lab. If you have an app, calendar, or spreadsheet tracking your cycles, you will have data that is more reliable than your doctor's lab test. The frequency of short cycles will tell a clearer story than the test.

Both Carole and Patricia tracked their cycles after we met, so they were clear about their Transition status. "No matter what my PCP told me about age or getting my hormone levels tested to confirm, I knew I was in the Transition," Carole said in my office. "Having that knowledge helped me remain open to options for getting help to address what was going on in my life." They both opted for HT, which helped tremendously with one of the biggest issues of the Transition: hot flashes!

Temperature Change and Biological Stress

Besides being the control center that regulates menstrual cycles, the hypothalamus is the brain organ that regulates systems as changes in the environment are detected. That includes heat and cold. The usual range of room temperature tolerance is plus or minus five to ten degrees Fahrenheit, beyond which the biological stress system sends an alert, pushing us, through shivering or sweating, to put on a sweater or to take it off. Temperature variation is such a reliable source of biological stress that for decades researchers have used it in their studies to measure the stress response. They may plunge a subject's hand into near-freezing water. They may shoot burning heat through a wire attached to the sensitive skin on the inside of the wrist. Either way, the sudden shift outside the normal range triggers a biological stress reaction to threat.

Nobody understands what the mechanism is yet, but during the Transition and sometimes well into the Upgrade the range of ambient temperature variation the hypothalamus can tolerate shrinks dramatically. This is called thermoneutral zone narrowing. There is some question as to whether this is due to a reduction in estrogen and progesterone making the hypothalamus hypersensitive to temperature. But here's what this means on a practical level. You are comfortable in your chair by the window in the early morning with your coffee or tea, content with the regularity of a ritual that has begun your day for decades. As the sun comes up, light pours into your room. You smile, anticipating the comfort of the warmth. Instead, irritation arises, followed by a surge of annoyance and a flush of heat from deep inside the core of your upper body that spreads outward over your neck and face, reaching your fingers and toes. If you took your temperature with a thermometer, it wouldn't register as a fever, but you might turn red or sweat or both. Bottom line: While everyone else feels perfectly comfortable, you'll want to swear like a sailor.

More than 80 percent of women experience hot flashes. They can last for a minute, five minutes, even half an hour. You might feel heat, sweating, flushing, chills, irritation, rapid heartbeat, and anxiety. Transgender men on hormone blockers to halt female puberty also experience hot flashes—the hormone blockers mimic menopause. This phase can last four to five years.

"The blow-dryer and humidity from a shower became my sworn enemies," says Carole. "If I had to do hair and makeup, I stood naked and barefoot on a cold floor. Sometimes I had to put cold packs under my feet. Even if the humidity in the bathroom cleared, the sheen of sweat on my face kept me from being able to apply makeup." I know what she means. I gave up everything but a little lipstick and blush. Patricia won't wear a scarf or socks in the winter anymore. "If I can't get my feet cool and my neck free, I will sweat the minute I come in off the street to a heated building."

While on the surface of things, we are talking about garden-variety hot flashes, what science hasn't paid attention to is the biological stress at their foundation. Think about what it means if temperature variation, one of the biggest natural stressors to the body, becomes intolerable to the hypothalamus. Through no fault of her own, constant, normal one- or two-degree room temperature fluctuations can mean a woman in the Transition and even in the Upgrade is living in a perpetual state of biological stress.

Sleep is the body's chance to reset and recover. But heat intolerance means that hot flashes may interrupt sleep during the Transition. Women tend to be too stoic about this. However if you are waking up twice or more during the night, you won't enter REM, and you won't get the rest you need.

Lack of sleep brings serious consequences to mood, ability to concentrate, metabolism, and the health of the heart. For more than 50 percent of women, this kind of distress can last between four and seven years or more after their final period. Though not troubled much by them, Ceci experienced occasional hot flashes into her late seventies. For me, as happens for many women on some form of HT, they went away when I started wearing the estrogen patch.

Estrogen stimulates the brain's production of the chemicals serotonin, dopamine, and endorphins—the brain's major contributors to well-being and feelings of joy. When those chemicals are lowered, they also bring down norepinephrine, which in turn reduces the ability of the brain's hypothalamus to tolerate heat. It was thought for many decades that estrogen therapy alone was needed to address the lowering of norepinephrine. New research is showing that progesterone might also mitigate the brain's estrogen withdrawal and help reset the temperature tolerance range of the hypothalamus. You just might be able to enjoy that cup of coffee in your sun-filled kitchen again.

Alarm Bells!

There is a little organ in the brain called the insula whose job it is to ping the body's various systems with one question: Are you okay? Before the Transition, on most days, unless you are stressed or sick, the response comes back *yes*. If there is even a small variation in the body's systems, and the response to the are-you-okay ping is *I'm not sure,* then the biological stress system kicks in. Adrenals turn on and cortisol and adrenaline heighten our ability to search for answers, if we are conscious of the stressor. Some of the time, biological stress turns into unconscious anxiety. The biological stress system of brain and adrenals is triggered by the insula's not getting the answer it expected, leaving us with a destabilizing brew of cortisol, adrenaline, and wildly fluctuating signals for follicular estrogen and progesterone. Carole's feelings of instability and her lack of her former resilience was an expression of these neurochemicals.

If you have any worries in your life at this time, like relationship, health of family members, financial concerns, or worry over a child, it's like pouring a geyser of gasoline on an already-burning fire. The biological stress response is in a constant state of alert. It's no wonder that if your husband, your teenager, or a close friend looks at you wrong, it will register as a five-alarm fire. Normal levels of cortisol can heighten our alertness to learning and can bring a little excitement to the day. Even before the Transition, too much cortisol can cause trouble with focus and cognition. The constant flow during the Transition sets the stage for brain fog and confusion. One patient of mine described her wild swings as having scrambled brains. She reported feeling uneasy, moody, and hyperalert yet at the same time having difficulty thinking clearly. "I had all this energy," she said, "but I couldn't harness it. I couldn't stay focused. It was like being a racehorse at the starting gate, ready to run yet unclear about which direction to take off in."

The neurohormones from the ovaries and adrenals are just about the most powerful influencers on the mind the female body has. Waves of wild emotion, out-of-proportion anger, irritability, and intense sadness can be reactions to a drop; overexcitement and agitation can be pushed by a surge of estrogen or progesterone in response to the pituitary's demand for more. In a *New Statesman* article, columnist Suzanne Moore wrote of her own transition, "I don't really have the mood swings that some talk about. I have just the one mood. Rage."

The choreography between the brain and ovarian hormones—estrogen, progesterone, testosterone—and the brain and adrenal hormones—cortisol, adrenaline, and DHEA, which converts into estrogen and testosterone—are treated by doctors as two separate systems. But they are happening in the same body and clearly impact each other. If you are having cortisol and adrenaline surges because of stress—and anybody alive experiences stress—on top of estrogen and progesterone glitches during the Transition, this can be experienced as a powerful emotional meltdown and/or an intensification of hot flashes. Combine an estrogen drop with life stress great or small, and you have confusion, destabilized mood, sleep problems, and memory problems.

It doesn't have to be this way. There is a lot of help out there, and we need to speak up about it more often and more openly. I have helped Carole and Patricia and countless others to stabilize and weather the storm.

Three Stages of the Upgrade

So far we've been focused on the storm of the four stages of the Transition, because identifying the phase you're in helps you better understand what kind of help you'll need and when you'll need it. But when you've closed the window on the tumult, either naturally or surgically, here's what to look for.

Early Upgrade: Twelve months after your last period marks the beginning of this phase. Some women who still have a uterus and choose HT that mimics their natural cycles will continue to bleed monthly. For many others, it's a combination of joy over no more periods and shock in the face of a changing body. Resistance to the new reality marks this phase for many.

Middle Upgrade: This phase involves attempting to make friends with the new reality, exploring new life paths, feeling the pull of needing a break, and desperately wanting to heed the siren's call to disengage.

Full Upgrade: This stage means embodying the fullness of life, embracing the ups and downs, returning to purpose, speaking truth skillfully and effectively, and engaging as a mentor, pulled by the desire to find ways to leave humanity better than you found it.

I haven't included ages here, because I've seen some reach the Full Upgrade immediately and others remain in Early Upgrade for life. It depends on attitude and action.

————

Almost 90 percent of women turn to a healthcare provider for help during the Transition and the Upgrade. They're a big deal to go through. I want you to have the resources to address symptoms, so that you can think, work, sleep, function, and maintain healthy relationships. Armed with information about medicine, lifestyle, the benefits of staying active, healthy eating, and finally getting consistent sleep, we can teach our doctors how to help. Now that you have a better sense of whether you are in the Pre-, Early, Mid-, or Late Transition or in the Upgrade, you'll learn in the next chapter which actions are best taken to optimize the phase you're in. Knowledge is power; the ability to act upon it means the best is yet to come!

Navigating the Wilderness

Chapter 4

"I'm humming like a well-oiled machine these days," Patricia, fifty-five, told me during a session. I was overjoyed to hear this, as her journey over the previous five years had been a bit of an odyssey. Storms, whirlwinds, rocky shores, numbed-out sadness, drenched sheets, and sleepless nights. It was the kitchen sink of Transition experiences. I knew eventually she'd find her steadiness; the way through is different for everyone, and I wanted to know how she got there. "I'm thrilled, Patricia. Tell me what it's like now."

She sat up and smiled. "For the first time in my life, I can count on my mood. My energy is pretty steady, I'm sleeping better than ever, and I love not having to track cycles or mop up the damage after a hormonal explosion."

Patricia was steadier and more grounded than I'd ever seen her. When she first called me five years earlier, it was a different story. She was tearful, sweating, exhausted, bleeding heavily, and she was profoundly anemic. I was quite worried about her. She had just moved to a new city and was struggling to find a doctor who didn't have a four-month waiting list for an appointment.

"I called seventeen doctors," she reminded me. "I had huge uterine fibroids. I was weak and had heavy bleeding for several years. I had such bad anemia that I could hear the blood pumping in my ears. I couldn't drive myself anywhere, and a doctor friend of mine, when he saw my labs, was stunned that my ob-gyn hadn't been alarmed by how low my red blood cells were. She told me she wanted to continue to treat me with repeated ablations to control the bleeding." Having this procedure meant Patricia would have to go into the doctor's office, be sedated, and have the lining in her uterus burned. I remember her telling me that she would likely have to have this done several times a year. She didn't want to have to keep doing that. She didn't want to keep feeling so weak. She was tired of having to change clothes a few times a day, and tired of ruining sheets and mattresses from the heavy bleeding. She didn't want to have to deal with any more hormonal spikes and dips of the Transition. She'd didn't know how many more years her Transition would last, and she wanted it over with. She sought a complete hysterectomy.

Whether it happens surgically or naturally, the shutting down of the ovaries—making the uterus obsolete—has a direct impact on the brain. It doesn't mean the organs have to be removed. Everyone will feel differently about keeping or losing a body part, and there is no right or wrong decision. It's very, very personal, and surgery for some can feel like a violation of one's wholeness. But Patricia had specific quality of life and medical reasons besides the rough Transition she was going through. "My mother had a history of ovarian cancer at fifty-four," she told me, "and I didn't want the anxiety of quarterly ultrasounds to check my ovaries anymore. I had been doing it, as required by my ob-gyn, since my early thirties. At the same time, I couldn't wrap my head around repeated ablations and embolizations to stop fibroids from causing so much bleeding." She was nearly in tears as she repeated the story, the trauma still fresh.

For women, first transitioning out of childhood and then years later the transition of the Upgrade makes our essential sense of belonging fragile as we wonder if we are alone in what we are feeling and experiencing. Nobody posts the misery of their story on Facebook or Instagram, the golf-ball-sized blood clots that fall into the toilet, or our fears of destroying the upholstery of a friend's couch when Pre-Transition-sized tampons and pads fail. Those who were early or late with their Transition, just as those whose periods started earlier or later than their group, feel left out, with nobody to talk to, no one to validate their experience. Exposing that you are feeling depressed, perpetually exhausted, and in the grip of wild mood swings can feel like you'd be putting relationships, friendships, or career at risk. But the opposite is true. The best thing we can do is talk to others and find the helpers who will hear you. We are here.

Patricia came out of her isolation and asked for help. Eventually her ob-gyn agreed to a hysterectomy and then connected her to a colleague who practiced functional medicine. It took a couple of years, but they got her hormonal cocktail right. She was now on a combination of estrogen, DHEA, and progesterone. She applied a topical estrogen and DHEA in the morning to help with energy, and the progesterone a couple of times a week in the evening to calm and help her sleep. I was witnessing the results in the big warm smile emerging on her face.

To be clear, the Transition and the Upgrade take place almost exclusively in the brain, but what happens to the ovaries and uterus has a direct impact on neurocircuitry. The ovaries make or trigger the production of hormones that push and pull our reality and our mood. In fact, everything we first learned in the 1980s about lack of ovarian estrogen causing mood drops, memory problems, and brain fog came from women who had total hysterectomies without hormone replacement. They were the easiest to study because the complication of hormonal spikes from the ovaries was off the table. To optimize the Upgrade, some women will want or need surgery. But the cultural bias against it can be rough.

My transition was marked by heavy bleeding and some wild mood swings. In 2005 I was finishing my first book, *The Female Brain*, and training a new generation of doctors—who were and still are much more interested in the hormones around pregnancy and the postpartum period—at the Women's Mood and Hormone Clinic at UCSF School of Medicine. I had undergone several D & Cs (scraping of the uterine lining) and embolizations to deal with heavy bleeding from my large fibroids. I was taking the birth control pill to steady my Late Transition fluctuating hormones. I was tired and testy and at fifty-three ready to enter the Upgrade. Knowing what I know about this phase, I felt strongly that a hysterectomy with ovary removal and a post-op estrogen patch, without progesterone, would be the best way forward for me.

I was able to get the surgery, finally, after struggling to find a surgeon who did vaginal hysterectomies along with ovariectomy. Before the surgery I filled out the paperwork indicating I wanted everything removed, including the ovaries so that I wouldn't have to monitor for ovarian cancer. I knew I didn't need a cervix for structural support and keeping it would mean yearly pap smears. So, after being asked repeatedly about my decision, I confirmed, "Yes, take it all out." The other thing I wanted was an estrogen patch to be put on in the recovery room. This is now standard procedure, but it wasn't back then. I knew from the literature and from many of my patients that if my body were surgically deprived of estrogen from my ovaries, that I would hit a wall of brain fog, hot flashes, sleeplessness, and exhaustion that I couldn't afford. I had a book tour to do a few months later, and I needed to be able to function in an Upgrade, not a Downgrade.

It was a difficult time to be asking for hormone replacement because just three years earlier, in spring of 2002, a flawed report came out that, according to colleagues at National Institutes of Health (NIH), set women's health back at least twenty years. The incorrect story this report told made it nearly impossible for me, a doctor who specializes in women's hormones, to get the hormone therapy I wanted.

The Tale of Two Hormones

With estrogen receptors in every organ of the female body, the influence of this neurochemical is profound. In the 1990s, researchers discovered that estrogen is protective of heart health, brain health, bone density, and emotional balance. Studies at that time were clearly showing that estrogen HT lowers a woman's risk of dementia, heart disease, diabetes, and osteoporosis and so during the 1990s, more women than ever were experiencing the benefits. Ob-gyns, internal medicine docs, cardiologists, family medicine practitioners, and the newly board-certified functional medicine doctors were prescribing HT earlier, during the Transitions as opposed to waiting until the Upgrade.

Then the blow came in 2002, with the publication of the confusing and flawed Women's Health Initiative (WHI) report on the risks of using hormones in the Transition and the Upgrade. Warnings of early death, heart disease, stroke, and cancer spread like wildfire from the report's conclusions as the media picked up the story and ran with it. The WHI trial was shut down, and panic around early death spread among doctors and patients. HT came to a grinding halt.

By 2008, six years after the WHI report, only 5 percent of women in the Transition were taking HT. And while it focused on risks, the WHI report completely ignored the protective effect estrogen has on brain, bone, metabolism, vaginal, cardiovascular, and emotional health. Those benefits are real and that data predates the WHI report.

Twenty years later, in 2021 and 2022, indications are that some of the data were flat out wrong. For example, the study had left out a crucial piece of information about the participants who were on HT and had had a heart attack or stroke. These women *already had underlying cardiovascular health issues* when they started the study. Their diets, smoking habits, alcohol intake, and lifestyles were not factored in. Additionally, at an average of sixty-four years old, they were fourteen years past their last period when they started HT. We knew then and know now that the benefits of HT are reaped if it is begun within five years of the Upgrade. We knew then and we know now, that if you wait to start for ten years or more, HT can be harmful.

The WHI report also indicated a marked increase in the risk for breast cancer for women taking HT, but again their data were flawed. There were women in the study who had undetected cancer before starting HT and some were BRCA positive, meaning they carried the gene giving them a 70 percent chance of developing breast cancer. The researchers should have eliminated these women from the data, but they did not. Even so, when the data was reanalyzed, the absolute risk of breast cancer after 5.6 years of combined estrogen and progestin therapy in the study was increased by less than 0.1 percent. But the impact of the report was real. Women stopped taking estrogen, and doctors stopped prescribing it.

With the massive reduction of women taking HT, if it were really harmful to the health of postmenopausal women, we should have seen an improvement over the two decades following the release of the WHI report. If there were indeed a risk of stroke from HT, the number of strokes in 2021 should be much lower than the number in 2002, when so many women stopped taking HT. But the rate hasn't changed. Not even a little bit. It puts a spotlight on the question as to whether or not HT causes strokes in women at all. And meanwhile, for two decades, women have been suffering symptoms of sleeplessness, sadness, confusion, and brain fog that could have been remedied by HT.

Increasingly, as doctors recognize the problems with the WHI report, the knowledge around HT that went dark for twenty years is being retrieved, and many have quietly resumed studying and prescribing hormones again. Disagreement around HT remains. The North American Menopause Society (NAMS) and the American College of Obstetricians and Gynecologists (ACOG) no longer oppose prescribing it, but the American College of Physicians (ACP) has produced statements claiming the risks of cancer and other diseases are too high. New studies are emerging at a rapid pace, and the bottom line consensus in 2021 has changed again: If women start HT around the time of the Late Transition and the Early Upgrade, the risk of cardiovascular issues is not only very small, there are cardiovascular and bone protective benefits of HT, especially from estrogen. Cognitive benefits of estrogen also look promising—it may be a factor in preventing dementia in women.

What always troubled me about the WHI report is that *quality of life* for women was taken off the table, as though getting enough sleep and balancing and improving mood had no contribution to overall health. Patricia felt she was living proof that it saved her mental health and her ability to earn a living. Without at least a low dose of HT, many women feel deep sadness and a profound lack of energy. Nearly 90 percent of all women have experiences that are troubling enough during the Transition and Upgrade to seek medical help. For some women, sadness can be a bigger health risk by far than that posed by HT.

If I'm feeling down, whether the cause of the sadness is a life event or low estrogen, I know from research, from decades of work with patients, and from my own experience that self-care will not be at the top of the priorities list. Feeling down never made me want to exercise, even though I am fully aware that moderate cardio four times a week is at least as good as, if not better than, SSRIs (antidepressants) for improving mood. If I am consistently sad, I am less likely to seek social connection, which has a proven impact not only on sadness but on cognition and longevity.

The New Medical Landscape

If you do decide to explore HT, like many, you'll probably start with the doctor you know best, your gynecologist. The benefit of partnering with this doctor is that likely you've known them for a long time, and the medications they use have FDA approval, which means solid studies, longevity of usage, and a treasure trove of information on how they impact your health. But for your ob-gyn or PCP to be of help, she will need to have added to her training like getting certified by the North American Menopause Society (NAMS). It's an entirely different area than what most ob-gyns are trained for. They are incredible at their specialty, which is pregnancy, childbirth, cancer detection, and surgical procedures. Their knowledge and skills center on the uterus, which is a muscle, and the ovaries. Yet it's the brain that is center stage during the Transition and the Upgrade. It's entirely the brain. For those out there who still need the low-pitched bellow of a man in order to hear this message and believe it, I give you the former ob-gyn and professor at University of Rochester School of Medicine James Woods. He's one of the few earlier gynecologists who decided to specialize in the Transition and the Upgrade because he recognized that he needed a knowledge base other than what he got in his training in obstetrics and gynecology. In his words, "[The *M*-word/Upgrade] is as different from obstetrics as surgery is from pediatrics." And because of his efforts, maybe we can forgive him for using the M-word.

The aftermath of the WHI report turned HT into a bit of the Wild Wild West. It led to trying to get estrogens via phytoestrogens in foods like soy, a hairball of an issue. Women with certain cancer risks can't touch it, and its high fat content means packing on the pounds. It doesn't help with hot flashes, vaginal dryness, joint pain, or brain fog either—phytoestrogens don't work on the brain or body in the same way that Premarin, synthetic estrogens, or bioidentical estrogens do. Herbal treatments like dong quai are entirely unregulated, and there are health risks to taking them as well. Dong quai can cause anxiety in some women. Black cohosh has been proven ineffective.

Bottom line is that I don't recommend trying to get your hormones replaced at the health food store. The best bet is seeking out responsible doctors prescribing FDA-approved HT or customized oral and topical so-called bioidentical hormones like estradiol, progesterone, DHEA, and others. They can track levels through blood and urine tests. Bioidentical hormones are manufactured to be the same structurally as our natural hormones. They are not considered to be better than other prescription forms—in some cases they are not FDA regulated and that can be dicey. But a good practitioner will do regular blood work to check your levels and prescribe hormones via what's called a 503A or 503B FDA-certified compounding pharmacy. You can find a list of qualified pharmacies on the United States Food and Drug Administration website. For some women who are sensitive to dose and sourcing, being able to easily customize is a good option. But it's easier, and probably safer, to try the standard medical approach first. I personally use an FDA-approved twice-weekly estrogen patch. Everyone's different—the best thing you can do is to become an observer in your own science experiment, so keep track of dosages and how you feel each day.

Finding Your New Sweet Spot

Not every woman is going to need to take hormones, but if you're having trouble functioning day-to-day, if your mood feels wildly out of control, or if there is a feeling of lifelessness that is not clinical depression, then HT might be a good road for you to take. Now that we know it's relatively safe, the risks are low, and it has protective benefits for the brain, heart, vagina, and bones, you can feel confident taking it with the help of your doctor.

You may ask, "Well what about breast cancer?" Taking estrogen plus progesterone for longer than five to ten years may cause a small increase in the risk of breast cancer. It's best to discuss your individual risk and genetics with your doctor. What I can tell you as of now is that if you take HT make sure to get an annual mammogram, keep your weight in the normal range, do moderate exercise, don't smoke, and stop drinking alcohol, since alcohol of any kind, including wine, doubles your risk of breast cancer. I wish I could tell you alcohol in moderation is okay, but the studies so far haven't broken it out that way. They show it as an all-or-nothing variable.

Keep in mind that the advice here is also not the bible on HT—it would be impossible to write that given the damage done by the WHI report and the fact that so much new research is emerging. The thinking is evolving by the minute. What I'm trying to give you, after studying the evolution of thinking around HT, is a snapshot of where we are now.

If you're going to start HT, research is showing that timing matters. If you start HT in the Late Transition and take it for three to five years after entering the Upgrade, then you will get those health benefits late into life even if you stop taking it. But if you wait too long to start, then HT can be harmful. Estrogen works well with healthy brain cells, or neurons. But if those neurons have been deprived of estrogen for too long and have started to age too much, then estrogen might even speed that aging process. The same is true of the cells in blood vessels and the heart. One study showed that this was the case in women who were sixty-five and older when they started HT with estrogen. But don't worry. If you've already missed that window, you'll find a ton of things you can do, especially through food, lifestyle, and exercise, that will protect your brain and heart. (See Chapters 6 and 11.)

If you are in the Early, Mid- or Late Transition, or Early Upgrade, then you can feel confident that there is safe hormonal help out there for you. Tell your doctor about everything you're going through, and that you want to give estrogen supplementation a try. The birth control pill might be right for you in the Pre- or Early Transition, and HT in the Mid- or Late Transition and Early Upgrade. And if you don't want to have periods or bleeding anymore, tell your doctor so she can adjust your hormone formula accordingly.

If you are in the Pre-Transition—experiencing body temperature regulation issues like having trouble cooling down from a workout but you are not yet having irregular cycles—then it's too early for estrogen supplementation. Raising estrogen alone at this stage can cause too much thickening of the uterine lining. If there isn't a steep enough monthly progesterone drop, that lining will continue to build, and you'll get breakthrough or heavy bleeding. Your doctor will need to use high doses of progesterone or need to scrape the lining out via D & C. Estogen supplementation at this time is just unnecessary.

Progesterone, which you'll need if you still have a uterus, can be calming or depressing, as most women know, because they've experienced PMS. You know what your cycling hormones feel like, and you also know that you can handle anything for a couple of days. But if you've been given progesterone in some form in order to control heavy bleeding and you notice you've got that weepy, cranky, foggy PMS feeling most of the time, it might be the progesterone. Talk to your doctor about changing form, lowering the dose, or other non-progesterone alternatives. If you do still have your uterus, your doctor may need to observe the uterine lining via ultrasound to track thickness, and you might need a quarterly dose of progesterone in order to flush it out.

If you are having hot flashes and are unable to sleep (more on this in Chapter 6), please don't feel like you have to muscle through without help. Small doses of estrogen (17-beta estradiol [oral 1 mg/day or transdermal 0.05 mg/day] or conjugated estrogen 0.625 mg/day) have been effective in eliminating hot flashes in 80 percent of women and can provide relief by reducing them in the other 20 percent.

Testosterone or, for some women, DHEA can help with libido and energy. If your husband is using a topical gel, you'll need much less than he takes, so don't borrow his!

It will be more important than ever to take good care of yourself while you're on HT because fitness, body fat, diet, and lifestyle can be a factor in whether or not you get the benefits. It's why I've got two chapters on exactly this. I want the neuroscience of health and well-being to be absolutely clear to you. And while studies are showing that obesity, smoking, and alcohol each erase the benefits of HT, remember that even three to five years of HT within the window of effectiveness has a lifetime of positive impact on bone and cognitive strength.

The Pill or HT?

"I had a really scary reaction," Patricia said of her struggle with the pill. "I blew up from bloat, I felt wildly testy, and when it didn't stop the bleeding, my doctor put me on a higher dose. When that didn't work, I started pure progesterone. It not only didn't stop the bleeding, I was catatonic, sobbing, on the couch. I have never been clinically depressed. But those chemicals incapacitated me. I couldn't think. I was completely unable to work, and I was in the middle of trying to start over in New York after my job ended. I had no energy, no zest for life and the consequences were life-altering. I was lucky I had savings to help get me through this time."

If you've started to have the irregular cycles and heavy bleeding of the Mid- or Late Transition, your ob-gyn might have suggested you take the pill. It's the go-to fix every doctor reaches for to stabilize cycles, control bleeding, and provide contraception any time during a woman's life, from a girl's first few years of menstruation to the Transition. The hormones of the pill take the ovarian follicle/pituitary/hypothalamus signaling system offline. If the brain senses enough progesterone and a low steady estrogen, it won't send out FSH or LH to push ovulation or build up the uterine lining. As the pill sends out a consistent signal, the pituitary and hypothalamus can relax. Under control of the pill the cycle becomes regular and the bleeding decreases. On the other hand, there's important information in those non-pill irregular cycles; being able to hear them is one of the Upgrade's greatest lessons in self-care. It can teach us to listen to what the body needs instead of muscling past a call to rest. Opening our ears to those needs becomes crucial to optimizing the Upgrade.

While not knowing when you are going to bleed is inconvenient, having irregular cycles in the Mid- and Late Transition isn't usually a big deal in terms of health. Often, there may be another cause, like biological stress that can result from life stress. Any stress can be intensified by irregular sleep, or inconsistent or excessive exercise habits—at this stage, more is not helpful and overexercising can kick off an explosion of stress hormones. The motto becomes exercise to exhilaration, not exhaustion. Every situation is different, but for many women, supporting the body with good habits and giving it time to find its homeostasis can put you back on track. But if heavy bleeding has been going on for a while, and is becoming incapacitating, that's another story.

There are over fifty variations of the pill. Each one has a different amount and combination of hormones. Doctors will typically try you on several to see what is most effective, starting with their best guess. When you are told you need a stronger pill to regulate bleeding, that usually means you will be getting a higher dose of progesterone. Some women can tolerate that. For many, they just feel rotten—bad mood, brain fog, trouble concentrating, feeling weepy, or flirting with the edge of clinical depression. The symptoms prompt many to quit. For some in the Transition, like Patricia, the progesterone in higher dose birth control is psychiatric poison.

More than 100 million women around the world take birth control pills, and shockingly little is known about the short- or long-term effects. Progesterone can be calming and settling, but if it's just a smidge off or the wrong type, it suppresses enlivening, ebullient connectivity of the brain. The science is becoming clear that progesterone from birth control pills is implicated in a tripling of suicide rates among women, with the highest numbers in teen girls who never had depression or anxiety before.

If there is a dramatic uptick in suicide rates among teen girls on the pill, which is mostly progesterone, to me, it's reasonable to extrapolate serious caution for women in the Transition who are put on progesterone. Worried about this consequence, I started asking the nation's leading experts if anyone was studying how to do better HT for women who had a variety of reactions to birth control pills or who had reactions to their own hormone fluctuations like premenstrual mood problems. I was told my question was excellent but there aren't any studies with good data. At the same time, between 1999 and 2010, the fastest growing rate of suicide was not white men. It was among women of all ethnicities around the age of sixty. Yet the phenomenon is not being reported nor is it being studied.

Like estrogen, progesterone is a potent neurochemical that can alter our mood or change our reality. If a doctor offers you a strong dose of progesterone in the form of a high dose birth control pill, an implant, a straight progesterone supplement either topical or oral, or a progesterone-infused IUD, make sure you can tolerate the neurochemical first. Before you get a device inserted, ask for an oral or topical (cream) prescription that would be an equivalent dose of progesterone and see what it does to your mood. Track it daily in a journal. Take it for at least three weeks before you decide about an IUD or implant. Please make sure you have a partner or close friend nearby to help you monitor your moods. And note that progesterone might reduce your sex drive.

Even if you had a hard time with a high dose of progesterone in the pill, you might do just fine with the much lower HT dose of progesterone in combination with estrogen. The only way to find out is to try it and to stay vigilant about mood and outlook. Keep a daily mood journal (see appendix, page 263) and note how pessimistic or joyful you feel for about three weeks. If you find that life sucks and everything is terrible, check your hormone doses with your doctor.

Be prepared to push back when an MD tells you that you shouldn't be feeling a certain way from a therapy. How you feel may be different from how a sister or a friend felt on the same medication, or after the same procedure. Everyone has a different experience, and to me, the patient is always right. Our job as doctors is to listen to an experience and see if we can translate that experience into medical terms that show us how to help her take the next right step. We have to learn to celebrate the messiness of individual differences. If you've tracked an experience in your mood log that clearly corresponds to the introduction of a new prescription and you're not feeling right, bring it up with your doc and make sure you are heard. You will know better than anyone what's right for you.

Switching from the Pill to HT

Susan, fifty-one, was taken off the pill for the first time since her late thirties, and her doctor suggested she stay off hormones. "I felt miserable. I begged to go back on." I helped Susan find a new doctor who had been quietly using HT for certain patients in spite of the WHI and other flawed reports that would emerge in its wake. In an off-the-record conversation, this doctor had told me, "The truth is many women do better with estrogen, and others don't need it. I find that the naturally occurring estrogen, 17 beta estradiol, and progesterone are a fine option for most of my patients." The doctor, age fifty-six, was taking it herself, and she wasn't the only ob-gyn I knew who was doing this. One study found that the majority of female ob-gyns who are in the Transition or Upgrade use HT on themselves even if they didn't recommend it to their patients.

How do you find out if going off the pill will be a problem for you? By going off the pill. For 20 percent of women, going off the pill isn't a big deal. But for the vast majority, if they go off the pill and are in or past any of the four phases of the Transition, it might wreak emotional and physical havoc. You can find yourself in horrible withdrawal as the pituitary, hypothalamus, and ovaries struggle to come back online. If you're between forty-eight and fifty-four, Early, Mid- or Late Transition, you can bet the restart is going to be glitchy as the brain, unplugged from any form of hormonal contraception, tries to reboot a faulty system in which there are likely already some power outages. As the system sputters back on, it can feel like you've gone crazy. It can be a WTF moment. Warn your partner first.

Remember that estrogen is an essential joy vitamin for many women, just as testosterone is for men. When estrogen levels crash, you may feel all the color, all the air, even your impulse to smile has suddenly vanished. You can feel bereft for no identifiable cause. The pill is four to eight times stronger than HT, so a straight switch is like giving up your smartphone for an old flip phone.

"When my new doctor suggested HT instead of the pill," Susan told me, "I balked. I thought, *that's for old ladies.* But she gave me a prescription for a very low HT dose. I didn't feel a lot better." Susan and I worked together with her ob-gyn to get it right. It's not always a simple switch to HT, but by increasing her HT dose, we could support Susan's Transition.

If you are of an age that puts you in Mid- to Late Transition and decide to shift to HT from hormonal contraception, you have to step the pill dose down gradually, otherwise you fall off a cliff. Lots of docs have learned to start with the higher HT doses, 1–2 mg of estradiol, which is still one-half to one-fifth of what's in some pills. On the other hand, if you have already started HT and your doctor wants to raise your estrogen levels to help your mood, libido, and to protect your bones, make sure they do it gradually. There is some evidence suggesting that topical creams and patches, like Vivelle, Climara, Alora, Estraderm, and Menostar, are safer than oral HT, and may have more flexibility in dosage. For those who have decided to use bioidentical topical creams, make sure you are rubbing it on a part of the body that can both absorb it easily and is far away from the breasts: the forearms, within three inches of the belly button, upper thighs, or for some forms, inserted with a vaginal applicator.

As far as HT goes, all I can tell you is what the data say and what I have experienced, what patients I've worked with have experienced, and what friends have gone through. For thousands of us, HT has helped. If you are frightened of it, I totally understand. I have the advantage of being a doctor with knowledge of the risks and benefits identified in research. I was able to make a decision decades ahead of where the thinking was because of the knowledge I had access to.

The most important thing is for you to recognize the impact of what you are taking has on you and to speak up. You and those close to you will know what is working and what isn't, what you can tolerate, and what pushes you over the edge. I encourage you to challenge your doctor, especially if you are sensitive to any substances. If you develop breast soreness or if you are beyond the Transition, are not on cyclic HT and develop breakthrough bleeding, speak up immediately to have your dose adjusted and your endometrium checked. If you're edgy, your estrogen may be too high. Above all, if you choose HT, make sure to do what you can to keep your risk factors for other diseases low.

SSRIs and non-HT Interventions

If you are suffering from hot flashes and cannot take hormones, SSRIs, antidepressants known as serotonin reuptake inhibitors, may be of help. They were first used on men suffering from hot flashes while undergoing hormone blocking therapy for prostate cancer. It turned out that the SSRI paroxetine—most commonly sold in the United States as Paxil—which was being studied in these men on Lupron (the hormone blocking drug) to treat sadness, also helped alleviate their hot flashes. As a result, they decided to test it on women having hot flashes during the Transition. Paroxetine at a dose of 7.5 mg turned out to be effective for some women as well, and so the drug was renamed and rebranded for women as Brisdelle in the United States. It received FDA approval in 2013 for treating hot flashes in women.

For Sarah, a film industry executive who was wary of HT, antidepressants turned out to be the perfect solution. "At the same time that I was going through the Transition, my boss, who had been a lifelong mentor and sponsor, retired. The woman who replaced him was edgy and explosive, and I needed to keep my balance if my career was going to survive. I had a hard time on hormones, so when my doctor mentioned an SNRI—antidepressants similar to SSRIs—Effexor/venlafaxine, to help me sleep, support my mood, and keep me even I said, 'Give me the pills!'" For her it worked like a charm.

Almost a quarter of women over fifty are on some form of antidepressant and while SSRIs work for some they may not be right for everyone. Tanya, a furniture maker living in Detroit who struggled with intractable melancholy, couldn't tolerate progesterone given to her during the Transition. She said it intensified her sadness. So, her psychiatrist began treating her hot flashes and melancholy with paroxetine. Tanya told me, "I felt like I had been brain damaged," she said. "While traveling in Europe for work, for the first time in my life I had suicidal ideation. I forced myself to go running every morning to keep from thinking about it. With the help of my doctor, I got off it, but it took me several years to climb out of that feeling and get back to myself. By the time I did, the Transition was over, and I was a completely different person. It took me a long time to catch up with myself and find my balance again."

Paroxetine can be effective, but it also has a long list of side effects that can be worse for some than the discomfort they are attempting to alleviate. These include, from the manufacturer's information: "anorgasmia, headache, fatigue, generally feeling unwell (malaise), lethargy, nausea, vomiting, increased dreaming/nightmares, muscle cramps/spasms/twitching, nervousness, anxiety, restless feeling in legs, or trouble sleeping (insomnia)." A new concern from studies is that paroxetine showed an increase in the risk for dementia, the very thing estrogen may protect against. It's not definitive, but there is enough smoke there to make us worry that it's indicating fire.

———————

I'm often asked what happens to the brain during the illness of depression. We know a bit about shifts in neurochemical processing, that the ability to make and utilize the body's natural feel-good neurohormones is interfered with. But what's really important to know is what those neurochemical shifts do to a person's reality. In the depth of their melancholy, they may find it hard to remember ever feeling any differently, even if you've known them to. Their brain circuits will not be able to access that former reality. As the outside world recedes, melancholy draws one ever closer to the siren call of suicidal ideation. It becomes almost a nervous system addiction. As patients recover, the death wish recedes, but for many it remains a persistent whisper. If this happens to you and lasts more than a month, reach out quickly to your medical team since help is available. And with new brain research on the effectiveness of cognitive techniques and medication, those emerging from intractable melancholy can come into a new relationship with their thoughts, to safely face reality.

For close to 60 percent of women, SSRIs can be effective in treating both depression and hot flashes. If you have full blown, clinically diagnosed depression, and your doctor recommends therapy and antidepressants, follow their advice. Estrogen, while for many can boost optimism and zest for life, does not treat severe depression. But the sadness that can accompany the Transition isn't always this more intense state of anhedonia, the lack of joy in clinical depression. It's often a temporary side effect of shifting hormones and a shifting identity; of feeling like we are becoming invisible at work and to the culture—to men and younger women all at the same time. Sadness might be a normal grief reaction. So maybe we need to find a way to better address grief.

The hard truth is that women are more at risk for depression in the Transition and the Upgrade. Somewhere between 45 and 68 percent of women in the Transition report more symptoms of depression compared with around 30 percent of women before the Transition. And if you've had a bout with depression before the Transition, you're two to three times more likely to have one during and/or after. So, protecting your state of mind is important. The evidence is clear that estrogen protects the brain, cognition, and mood. With my patients in the Mid- to Late Transition, and the Upgrade, if they are clinically depressed, I often prescribe a combination of HT, therapy, and SSRIs. We monitor their sense of well-being closely, together. And while it doesn't treat depression, there is reason to believe that, if taken early enough in the Transition, estrogen, for some women, may stop a long slow slide into clinical depression.

When Sadness or Low Energy Is Anemia or a Thyroid Issue

For the women who experience excessive bleeding during the Transition, it's very common to develop anemia. Patricia did, and I remember her telling me during a session that she was "okay as long as I didn't have to get off the couch!" It's no way to live, and if it goes on long enough, anemia can cause deterioration in cognition as the brain loses oxygen. So, make sure your doctor monitors your hemoglobin and hematocrit levels. And if you've stopped bleeding, have your red blood cell width measured as well. It will tell you whether or not your bone marrow has caught up with cell production. When it has, then you can get off the iron supplements.

The thyroid, a little endocrine gland at the base of the throat, produces hormones (T3 and T4) that have a direct impact on preservation of cognition, on metabolism, and on how energetic we feel. The neurohormone system in the body is deeply interconnected, and for many women, the thyroid can be thrown off by the hormone changes of the Transition. So, if your skin and hair are dry, you are tired all the time, and you can't think straight, ask your doctor for a thyroid checkup since women have ten times more thyroid disease than men.

Tracking Your Moods

"My husband is an engineer," said Patricia, "and he loves spreadsheets. During the Transition, he kept track of my cycles on his calendar. I kept track too, just so I would know when to start loading up my purse with equipment. But that he did it? I was super sensitive about that at first. In fact, I was outraged. It felt so judged because he was doing it to track my mood. But he saved me a bunch of times. I would feel one hundred percent certain that a friend was angry or that a colleague was insulting me, and I would start to gear myself up for a big confrontation. And then he would say, 'Darling, before you burn the house down, would you consider checking your calendar?' The first few times he did this, I shredded him for what felt like a lack of support. But then I saw he was right. I learned to wait it out. And now that I take HT along with DHEA, he knows when I've been skipping my DHEA since I don't want to be touched down there."

By this point in life, you probably know plenty about the way your mood sinks along with your hormones and vice versa. Starting or stopping hormones can have the same impact. Any time you make a change to the hormones you're taking, let someone close to you know about it. If your behavior or mood shifts, ask them to tell you. Mood shifts can be so powerful that you may not recognize it as a change. It will just feel like your reality. The scary thing about hormones—and for that matter any chemical we take—is that we often can't separate how they're making us feel from what is going on in our lives.

You don't have to make a spreadsheet like Patricia's engineer husband but do consider keeping a daily record when you start new hormones or medications. I like my patients to write it all down every day until we find the correct balance. (See appendix, page 263, for detailed instructions.) When you've charted what's going on for six to eight weeks, you can figure out what is going on and have data to help you adjust the dosage accordingly. With most of my patients, we find their new sweet spot after three to six months. With this kind of information in hand, you have a better chance of making it happen sooner.

No one can feel happy and focused all the time, but you deserve to have more good days than bad during the Transition and in the Upgrade. Your hormones can be an aid to this if you get the balance right. For some women, hormones may improve mood and memory and decrease irritability right away. For others it takes a few tries to get the balance right. The most critical thing about taking hormones is how they make *you* feel.

Balance

Homeostasis, the body's fight for balance, is often visualized as an inverted U-shaped curve, like the perky breast that once upon a time in our teens and twenties stood straight up even when you were lying down. Let's say that homeostasis is at the nipple level and for many years you probably hovered there. You knew what it felt like to be in your body, what the experience of your mind and life force felt like. As hormones shift in the transition, as they pull other neurochemicals with them that regulate sleeping, waking, biological stress, temperature variation tolerance, you get pulled off homeostasis. You end up on the downside of the curve instead of at the top. You feel off, not quite yourself because what you are experiencing in your own skin is not how you remember feeling. It's not how you remember the experience of who you are.

On top of that, you've gone for a checkup and gotten lab work done. After decades of perfect scores in cholesterol, inflammation markers, vitamin and mineral levels, suddenly everything is off. Your cholesterol had been 156 for decades and now it's 210. Your blood glucose was always low and now it teeters on the brink of prediabetes. Your blood pressure has always been 110/70 and now is 132/85. Your vitamin B and D are tanked out. The confluence of the Transition and age conspire to try to make you realize you are not twenty-five anymore. And that is a tough pill to swallow.

I want to reassure you that your out-of-whack numbers will settle, even if it takes a few years. The neurohormonal wildness of the Transition causes unhealthy inflammation in the body and brain, and that will settle with time, maybe HT, diet, and lifestyle adjustments. You will find your sweet spot again, but it won't be the same one you have been used to. How you experience homeostasis will never be the same. If you can make friends with your new sweet spot you might find it's even better. It requires more patience than you ever thought you would have but I promise, you will find that patience through care for yourself, and it will pay off.

I can't deny that this is a risky and difficult time. Don't make big decisions when you're in the thick of it. Take life planning in chunks. If you are in any of the Transition phases and feel like you want to make a dramatic change, wait one month, then three months, six months, even eighteen months, until you feel more steady and clear. And you will—homeostasis is out there, whether it happens for you naturally or with the help of a medical practitioner. Like a whirling top that's hit a bump in the floor, you might wobble like crazy for a while. But you will recover a new, stable, and effortless spin.

Renewal: Your Brain in Search of a New Reality

Chapter 5

"Honey, I wouldn't look hot in this ever again, even if I could lose the weight," sixty-six-year-old Ceci said to Carole's daughter Dawn. She pulled a tiny, sexy dress out of the closet and gave it to the twenty-two-year-old woman. "It's a dangerous one, so be careful! I remember walking into a room and all the men's eyes were on me. I was wrapped around my first husband's arm when two guys walked over together and tried to pick me up," Ceci said with a laugh. There's not a hint of regret in her voice.

Ceci had first met Carole, Dawn's forty-seven-year-old mother, fifteen years earlier, when the younger woman had come to her for advice. Carole quickly adopted Ceci as a mentor, and before long they became close friends. Dawn had just graduated from college and was about to start work. I was visiting Ceci when Dawn and Carole showed up for a quick celebration and a treasure hunt in Ceci's closet.

Carole knew how important Ceci's looks had been to her and wondered why she didn't seem sadder about how her body and life had changed. Carole herself was dreading the future and for now remained happily in denial that she would ever not be skinny. "You think you will never have baggy arms or watermelons for breasts," Ceci said to Carole, "but say hello to both. Yours will probably be worse. There's nothing to do but embrace being healthy on the inside, and celebrate: NO MORE PE-RIODS!!"

Carole was ogling Ceci's vast collection of anti-aging products laid out on the bed, a pile of high-end skin-care products and makeup received over the years as perks for being in the fashion industry. Ceci noticed. "Take them all, Carole. I don't use them anymore. I don't want one single package in my house that insists I have to anti-age. It pisses me off just looking at them. It took me a long time to remember what I know from the industry—that anti-aging is the marketing response to the fear of young women. It's Dawn and her friends who are the ones freaking out about wrinkles. They are getting their faces sliced up and injected. Not me!"

Ceci is right, though it seems counterintuitive that the vast majority of women undergoing cosmetic procedures are well under fifty. "For a long time I was tortured over losing my looks," Ceci said, continuing her diatribe. "And I remember the torture of trying to hide my age. I'd forget who I told what year I was born or graduated college, and I was always worried I'd be outed. I thought it mattered whether or not my colleagues thought I was ten years younger than I was. But then one thing got super clear: If you get into a fight with reality, who's going to win? I'd been holding on to an idea of who I was and how my looks and my job defined me. No matter how evolved we think we are as women, this stuff is deep in our nervous system. It was a big, big struggle. Don't let anyone kid you about how hard it can be. Once I allowed myself to grieve my old life and my old self, things got much simpler. Now that I am proud of every wrinkle on my face and every year I've lived, I don't have to worry about what I say when someone asks my age. I tell them straight up."

Ceci paused, though, at the memory of the hormonal roller-coaster ride of the Transition. She'd been reluctant to talk about it when Carole had asked. But I was used to drawing women's stories out. After some hesitation, Ceci talked about how it had felt like crazy people were playing a wild tennis match with her brain and moods. With the ups and downs of hormones came the torture of the insula, the part of our brain that scans our body systems to confirm health and check self-image. Beginning with the first transition to the teen-girl brain, the insula compares what we look like to what others look like, influencing how we think about ourselves in relation to others. *Do I look as good? Can I look like that? Would I rather look like someone else? What's my style?* It's the brain area for feeling disgust at the gap between expectation and reality.

For many women the mental and emotional patterns that recruit the insula can set us up for a lifetime of obsession with weight and appearance. But other than making sure she gets healthy fats for her brain and stays away from too many energy-draining carbs, Ceci decided to ignore the insula's prods and stopped dieting after the Transition ended. She discovered what many women figure out after the Transition: that as estrogen drops, your metabolism changes. Eating carbs will just stimulate the brain to want more and to squeeze more insulin out of your pancreas, so carbs make your blood sugar spike and drop much more dramatically. If we keep feeding the brain's craving for carbs, diabetes is more easily triggered; the resulting inflammation can damage joints, arteries, and cognition. To keep her energy even throughout the day, Ceci accommodated her brain's new metabolic needs by feeding it more lean protein and healthy fats. For Ceci, as for many women, it was trial and error until she found the right blend.

"Now that I'm not cycling up and down every month, things are so much more peaceful. I feel comfortable in my own skin in a way I never did in my life. I feel so confident, so strongly rooted in who I am that I wouldn't trade a flat stomach, a wrinkle-free face, or even joint pain for the suffering of those years. My body is what it is. And I get to see happiness in your daughter's face at taking home some great clothes," she told Carole, smiling. "And the best thing about doing business with men is that since they're not trying to figure out how to get me into bed, they finally listen to what I have to say. They are taking me seriously in a way they never did."

Ceci had been through tremendous shifts in her career in the fashion industry, and in her personal life. She had three kids, all grown, the middle one a daughter, Stephanie, who had had a hard time getting her life started. A college dropout, she'd been unable to keep steady work, and

Ceci lived daily with obsessive worry and stress about whether or not Stephanie would find her way and be able to take care of herself. While she loved her craft, her corporate job had always been a source of stress. Ceci had been a textile designer for one of the most prestigious fashion houses in the world, but by the time she hit her late thirties, she had started feeling a pervasive anxiety. "I was having trouble sleeping. Something was making me deeply insecure. It took a long time for me to figure out what it was. And then one day it dawned on me. Every woman I knew who was a bit older than me was getting canned. It started happening in their forties. It didn't matter what industry, and it barely mattered how successful they were. Publishing, fashion, finance, TV, real estate, PR. Some were making it to their midfifties, but most of the women I know who worked for other people were being let go. I suddenly realized that I had a shelf life."

It's not a surprise that Ceci didn't recognize the source of her anxiety right away. Not only do we have an epidemic of it in America, with nearly one-fifth of the population reporting an anxiety disorder, but we now marshal every possible distraction to keep from feeling the discomfort. It's understandable that we'd reach for a smartphone, the TV, a glass of wine, food, anything other than the brain's experience of dread. In times of threat, the body is flooded with stress hormones that can make us go cold, our hearts feel like they are pumping out of our chests. Alertness is intensified. Our hands and feet can go numb as blood rushes to our muscles and brain. If the feeling becomes chronic, if we live with it all the time, then not only does anxiety become a disorder, but we are at higher risk for heart disease, diabetes, cancer, depression, dementia, and more.

But not all anxiety is bad, and research is supporting the truth of Carl Jung's admonition that with any negative state, "the more you resist, the more it persists." If we can be present to the message of anxiety, it can be a warning of real danger, like what happens when we are followed out of a grocery store late at night into a dark parking lot by a person with bad intentions. That is a strong signal, and fear is part of what helps us respond in those moments with potentially lifesaving actions, like returning to the store and asking for an escort or calling someone for help. Signals are there to get the brain to engage the problem-solving abilities of the prefrontal cortex. If we try to circumvent that call for engagement because a feeling is uncomfortable, we could be ignoring important information coming from deep within our own brains.

Dawn and Carole gathered up their bounty, a part of Ceci's former self she was consciously shedding, and took it home. Ceci and I headed out for coffee together. We were new friends—she'd just joined a meditation group I've been part of for twenty-five years. I was curious about her life and her decision to become an entrepreneur, a path many women in the Upgrade take. "When I was in my twenties and thirties," she told me as we sipped our drinks at Cafe Roma, overlooking the San Francisco Bay along Bridgeway in Sausalito, "I remember seeing older women packing their offices to leave. I didn't give it a second thought consciously, other than a passing feeling that they had lost their crispness and it was time to go. But looking back, I started having trouble sleeping after about four or five of them left within a few months of each other."

Ceci paused, remembering how hard it had been to stay alert at work, to keep her energy up when she was sleeping about three hours a night, how whacked her emotions felt. "Every morning I woke up terrified that that day at work would be my last," she continued. "I had no idea what I would do without my job and my identity."

In retrospect she acknowledges that the perceived chronic threat created a distortion field that contributed to the already-high tension at home with her daughter. Threat arising from lack of trust at work makes it difficult to develop real relationships everywhere else in our lives, and she and her husband had several tough years. Our brain is on alert all the time and not calm enough to truly incorporate or build friendships into our circuits. "It felt like a game of *Survivor*," she said. "You could make temporary alliances as long as we held some utility for each other. But as we all got closer to the prize, the path narrowed. You never knew who was going to push you aside in order to leap ahead." Hormones like adrenaline and cortisol are released in response to threat and are great in the short term for enlivening our focus and for inspiring great ideas. But over time, they take their toll and produce the opposite effect. "With all that drama at work," Ceci continued, "I just couldn't be as creative. My ideas weren't good anymore. I was having trouble being fast on my feet. I thought it was just age. What I saw happening to other women was starting to happen to me. I was losing my edge."

"Did it ever occur to you," I asked, "that losing your edge was not necessarily a function of age?"

"Not at first," she replied, "but later, when I had a chance to rest and heal, my mind came roaring back. Once I got away from a threatening environment, my brain got creative again."

It makes sense biologically. Cortisol, the hormone released when we are under pressure, can be friend or foe, depending on the duration and the amount. Women in the Upgrade have a higher cortisol reaction than before the Transition. Cortisol boosts our memory and our interest in learning when it's being released in the right amount. But if we get too much for too long, it kills memory cells.

"So what did you do?" I asked, riveted by her familiar story. I have heard variations of this story from my patients and from my friends. First we face a glass ceiling that keeps us from rising. And then we fall off the glass cliff. We live in an ageist society, and there is no doubt that all older people face discrimination in the workplace. But statistics show that women are aged out of their jobs as much as ten to twenty years earlier than men, depending on the industry.

"I gave up first class for a middle seat," Ceci exclaimed, borrowing a line from Laura Mercier cofounder Janet Gurwitch, who talks about leaving a plum job at Neiman Marcus to start the line of cosmetics that catapulted her to entrepreneurial stardom.

Ceci had an idea for her own company too. She'd been thinking of producing a flattering and more forgiving line of stylish activewear. But starting over in midlife wasn't easy. Where she'd had entrée into any office she wanted while connected to a multinational corporation, doors were no longer opening so easily. With the corporate perks gone, she was traveling around the country on a budget to pitch her new line, using money she'd saved for retirement to fund the new company. "When anxiety about that hit," she said, "I had to use my own brain's cognitive power to remind myself that I was making an investment, that I was betting on myself. If it weren't for the emotional support of my friends, I never would have gotten it off the ground. I nearly gave up a dozen times."

Ceci's journey to entrepreneurship is an increasingly common one among women in the Upgrade, from restaurant workers to executives. When the doors to employment close, those who can are paving their own roads by starting businesses themselves. "A very forthright executive coach was the one to wake me up," Marta, a fifty-four-year-old tax consultant, told me at her appointment. "She flat out said nobody was going to hire me at the level I was used to, and that the sooner I started my own business the better. Building a client base was really hard, and at first I was making a fraction of my former salary. There were so many times I thought I would end up on the streets. But eventually things started working. There is an extraordinary talent pool filled with women who've been aged out of corporations or pushed out because of still having young kids at home, and I am contracting out excess work to them. I can't even believe who I'm getting to partner with on projects, and how much I'm learning from the people I've hired." Her brain had kicked back in in full force.

Marta and Ceci have become part of a significant economic statistic. In the growth of the economy nearing the second decade of the twenty-first century, it's women who are the biggest drivers of job creation. From 2015 to 2016, women started businesses at double the rate of men. As of 2017, companies formed and led by women performed twice as well as those formed and led by men and were responsible for the creation of tens of millions of jobs. Of those female-led companies, the majority of the founders were over forty-five. In a May 2019 article for *Forbes*, Kevin O'Leary of *Shark Tank* talked about his preference for companies run by women. He said that while those led by men meet their targets 65 percent of the time, women have a much better record, meeting financial targets 95 percent of the time. The same article cites research showing that female-led companies are better for employee well-being, especially in the troubling area of engagement at work, where Gallup polls show that 70 percent of employees feel a lack. A lifetime of experience brings the knowledge that fuels success. And a lifetime of facing moments that bring us to our knees means women in an optimized Upgrade can live with uncertainty in ways that the untested among us cannot. We have built a brain that is more resilient under fire.

. Early in the growth of her business, Ceci had to sue to collect what she was owed from a large retail chain. "If they didn't pay me," she said, "I was going to go broke. It happens to a lot of people in the clothing business. You spend most of your time as a debt collector. But this one was a whopper that I couldn't absorb. I had to recover the money, or at least a significant portion of it. There was a moment when it didn't look good, where the other side was burying my lawyers in papers and we were starting to miss dates. I was overwhelmed by fear, and for the first time I wasn't sure if the feeling of powerlessness would actually kill me. It was clear that if I remained in this state it was going to seriously damage my health. I remember deciding to stop fighting it and let the feeling take over. I am not religious, but I prayed to all the forces in the universe for help. I wasn't asking that some magical being swoop in and rescue me. I didn't believe that was possible. But I was asking for the ability to be at peace with whatever happened. That if I lost everything, if I was out on the street, that I would be as okay with it as anyone could be." Luckily, Ceci wouldn't end up losing anything. Her lawyers were able to resolve the situation a few days later, but the emotional breakthrough meant that the hard stuff wouldn't ever again shake her up the way it used to. That moment of life bringing you to your knees and coming out with your balance is a sign of the Upgrade, as your brain circuits are primed for resilience.

Centering, feeling at home and at ease in a new reality, is a gift of the Upgrade. For the first time since childhood, many women have the experience of being released from competing agendas—the deep yearning of your authentic self and the reality and behavior driven by the fertility cycle. Hormones are there to shape priorities and to try to force you to act, to make sure you feel intimacy and connection with partners and children. It can feel like it's against your will. The intense estrogen spikes of the Transition can overwhelm the mind with obsession, pushing many women to repeat the habits—like attraction to bad boys—of their teenage years. The intense drop-off at the end of an estrogen spike can leave us so bereft of connection, attraction, and sex drive that we crawl into bed and turn off the phone.

At the same time, I don't want to ignore the fact that the fear of ending up impoverished is the number one threat that haunts older women in America; it is provoked by a signal that is real. While women carry 78 percent of the unpaid caretaking burden, we are, over the course of our careers, making 60 to 70 cents on the dollar compared to men. The wage gap is not the only contributing factor. Unequal pay combined with years of unpaid caretaking, in which women may not have the chance to work outside the home, means we have fewer resources as we age. Because we do not work outside the home for as many years as men do, our contributions to Social Security and retirement funds are lower, making the wealth gap all but uncloseable. Since 1990, divorce rates for couples over the age of fifty have doubled. So if we end up single in the second half of life, and we weren't able to work outside the home for much of our lives, many of us will be trying to survive on a $600-a-month Social Security check. While women like Ceci and Marta were okay—they had savings, and they'd been able to contribute to Social Security during their long working lives—most women after the Transition are not anywhere near financially independent. Knowing this financial reality opens the door to understanding why so many stay in difficult marriages and mimic their husband's attitudes, even those that are clearly misogynistic. Disagreement might mean being cut off from food, clothing, and shelter in old age.

Ceci had financial means, independence, and choices. Her new company not only got off the ground; it exploded. She eventually sold it and used the money to start her own venture capital fund. She focused on funding and mentoring and sponsoring young women, helping them take charge of their financial destiny by planning for the day when they would have to clear their own path. Relying on a corporation to provide employment for the rest of their lives just wasn't a realistic path anymore.

We Are So Much More Than We Have Been Taught to Believe

"It took a long time for me to realize that I actually have something to offer younger women." Ceci had rented a suite of offices in a quasi-open collaborative work space with other entrepreneurs in creative sectors. "They pop in whenever they have a problem," she continued. "I still don't feel like a grown-up myself, so I missed the cues at first, when they started coming around asking questions. Then I remembered having done the same at their age. I had so many older women friends during my twenties and thirties that one mentor called me a 'wisdom junkie.' It's finally dawning on me that they see me as I saw my mentors and sponsors, someone with hard-won wisdom. I keep being surprised by the fact that I often do have real answers to their big questions."

The idea of wisdom is daunting, and not something we connect with easily as women. I know from my own experience. The wildness of the Transition to the Upgrade can make us feel like moody teenagers, constantly regressing and misbehaving, feeling out of control. For most of us, that period of time doesn't feel like the budding of wisdom. It can feel more like all our brain's good qualities are being drained.

By the time you reach your late forties or fifties, you've been through a mountain of experience. You've traversed the turbulent teens, when you were trying to figure out who you were; the unpredictable twenties, as you struggled to find your way in the world; the buckle-down thirties, when you were trying to implement your life plan; and the juggling forties, when you were living the life you'd made for yourself—for better or worse. What's next? This is the big unanswered question.

Women in developed countries are living on average into their mid-eighties and beyond. The Transition can occur anytime in your forties or fifties. Medicine and developmental psychology have lumped what follows for women into one big post-*M*-word category. That's thirty to fifty years unmapped, unexploited, unaccounted for. There are no phases defined, no transitions delineated other than death. It's another reason I refuse to use their word.

I am here to signal to your brain that you are just getting started in becoming who you're meant to be.

Oh, Louann, no. I'm done. I'm tired. I just want to relax! I hear you. Women often feel burned out at this stage. We've been holding up our worlds for a long time—kids, career, caretaking, house maintenance. Taking breaks is fine. Everybody needs them. But I want to ask you to question the feeling of being *done*. What is it you are really done with? Is it something specific, or is it really as global as it feels? After a lifetime of earning less, working harder, being the one responsible for the caretaking, it's normal to feel *done*. But before quitting a job or a long marriage, make sure you have clear answers. Running away before you know what you're running toward can be a big mistake at any age but especially now. Make sure you know what you want. And consider that you might need a sabbatical, some downtime to reflect.

The flip side of this question is our vision for the future. At this moment it is time to ask ourselves the same question we asked in our teens and twenties: What do you want your life to look like now? Is it really one long beach vacation or series of art classes? Is it a new load of caretaking of aging parents, spouse, and grandchildren? Is it being saddled with the family home, which now feels like an albatross? Or is it a new career, a new adventure, a sense of delight that comes with having a beginner's mind? I want you to meet this time with joy, not with regret. I've heard too many of those stories.

Ching was born in San Francisco in the late 1920s. Her story is of another generation, but the expression of not having lived the life she wanted is one I've heard many times in my office. "I always loved America," she said during our third session. "But when my family made the money they planned to earn through trade, they took us all back to China when I was ten. I hated it." Ching had come to see me after having a small brain-stem stroke. We were trying to get her mood and ability to sleep, which had been disrupted by the stroke, back on track. Normally quiet and hard to draw out, she burst into tears and the words came pouring out: "I didn't do anything I wanted to do with my life. I wanted to go to college. I wanted to have a career. I wanted to continue to learn. I was teaching English when World War II hit, and I rode out the war in Macao, cut off from my family in Canton and Hong Kong, where the Japanese had landed. I had always dreamed of returning to America to go to college and go to work. I was a citizen from birth. After the war my parents agreed to let me go and sent me with an aunt to join my older brother, who was already in California. I was just getting settled when the communist revolution came. My family in China lost everything. My brother and I had to go to work to ransom my parents and siblings out one by one. We got my parents and one sister. I worked so hard at my brother's restaurant!"

I paused, waiting for this normally very composed woman to gather her thoughts. "So what about college?" I asked.

"I had to keep working. I finally got a job at a bank and was able to take care of my family. I spent my whole life taking care of everyone. It was hard. I was a woman, an Asian woman on top of that, and I was being underpaid. I knew it because I was part of an audit group. But I couldn't speak up because I would have lost my job if I did."

I tried to hold the space as her grief unfolded. "And now my body and brain don't work well enough for me to pursue any of those dreams. My life is gone and I did nothing I wanted to do with it."

Though Ching's story may sound extreme, many women face a version of this regret, but with some effort, the right help, and vigilance, this kind of deep sadness can be turned around. I worked with Ching to shift her focus to everything she did accomplish at work and with her family, and to remember how proud she was of her granddaughters, who were taking full advantage of so many opportunities by starting careers in molecular biology and environmental science. We talked about this in her sessions, got her sleep and mood back on track, and I gave her journaling homework to help her notice what went right in her life.

I am telling you this story because I want you and your brain to be prepared for the developmental phases of the Transition into a new identity, the early stages of the Upgrade, and the Full Upgrade, when we embrace and acknowledge the depth of our experience and develop a deep concern for feeding it forward, so that future generations have the benefit of our knowledge, taking it even further.

What I mean by a Full Upgrade is when post-Transition women act on the decision to grow into their full female potential. This includes independence of mind, strong compassion for oneself and others, and a view of life that embraces reality as it is, not how we wish it were. It's an act of volition, of personal agency. Passively riding out our later years in a fog of denial about old age and death is not optimized. It's not an Upgrade. It's giving in to the cloak of invisibility, of uselessness, the fossil concept of the *M*-word. A downgrade.

Growing into Wisdom

In my practice as a psychiatrist, I can track how someone is growing into and embracing their status as a wise old woman. In many cultures around the world, we are comfortable saying "wise old man." But when we swap out "man" for "woman," the phrase gets caught in our throats. When we were younger, we called older women cute, eccentric, little, sweet, loving, dear, but how often did we feel them to be wise? Though I knew instinctively that Grandma was the one who held the real secrets to life and relationships, it was still Dad and Grandpa who were running the show. Though women's wisdom may be revered by families and communities in Africa, in Asia, and among African American, Latino, and a few shamanic cultures, there isn't a single society in the world that has majority female leadership. If you break down leadership by the percentage of women holding the highest political offices and executive positions, and try to find a society that has pay parity over the life of a career, in which women have equal access by most measures to education and capital for success, there isn't a single country that comes close to a fifty-fifty power share. Women in the Upgrade can turn this around.

Men don't have trouble stepping into the role of counselor and sage. But for women it's one we too easily abdicate. "I just don't have anything to contribute," my patient Pauline said to me back in the mid-1990s. She was seventy-two, a well-informed, avid reader. She had worked as an executive assistant in between children. Pauline's sadness was palpable and heavy; I could feel its drag on my own emotions as we talked through her history. In psychiatry, we are trained to watch our own reactions as indicators to help us validate reactions our patients get from others in their daily lives. When I asked her if others felt sad when she told her story to them, she said they did, and she was afraid she would alienate her oldest friends if they really knew how unhappy she was.

We tried an antidepressant and weekly appointments. After a few months, not much had changed, and I was beginning to worry about whether I would really be able to help her. One day she arrived with a bit more energy, and I probed to see if I could figure out the source of the uplift. Pauline mentioned her granddaughter Michelle, who had just graduated from San Francisco State and was moving to Los Angeles for work. Michelle had come to Pauline for style advice, and from what I could see, it was a great choice. Understated and elegant, Pauline had impeccable taste even on a budget. While she and Michelle assembled Michelle's new wardrobe, they talked about family, past wounds, and fears for the future. Michelle was living a life Pauline had wanted for herself. "I wanted to work. I was in love with someone else, but my family pushed me into the marriage with George," Pauline said of her husband of fifty years. "Michelle was full of questions about her parents, about my life with her grandfather, about how she would survive in LA. I don't know why she thinks I have any answers that will help her. What do I know?"

I paused, thinking the interaction with her granddaughter was a good sign and wanting to encourage it. "So do you have plans to spend more time with Michelle?"

"We finished the job. She's ready to go," Pauline said. "I did what I can do. I can show someone how to buy clothes on a budget that will stay in style. I can throw a party. I certainly know how to keep up a strong front. But beyond that, what do I have to give?"

Michelle didn't see her grandmother the way Pauline saw herself. She persisted in the relationship, finding in Pauline a confidant, a safe place to turn when she was afraid about her own brand-new start in the world. "Grandma listens in a different way," Michelle would later tell me in a family session. "She didn't tell me to suck it up the way my mom and dad do. Well, sometimes she laughed at the things I was upset over and told me that in a few years they wouldn't matter, especially the guys I met who didn't call me back. That's a little irritating! But whenever I had trouble with someone at work or with one of my roommates, Grandma seemed to have had the same experience sometime in her life, and she told me what it was like for her. And she often told me the difference between how she handled things at my age and how, looking back, she would handle them given what she knows now."

When we are young, we learn language, concepts, and skills. In the Upgrade, we learn to see the wisdom that grows from the refining experience of success and mistakes, joy and tragedy. All of this comes as the brain settles into a regular pattern, less buffeted by hormonal waves, more able to absorb and integrate the lessons of the memories stored by the hippocampus into the cortex. By the time of the Upgrade, we have a mean, lean, problem-solving machine. Our job is to accept the challenge of embracing this role, to weave the strands of our experience into insight that benefits others. At the beginning of the Transition, the developmental phase plants the seed of wisdom by setting up the brain for resilience in a storm. You have this strength in your brain. One of your jobs is to water these and not be afraid of them, not be afraid of falling short of the wisdom that comes from having survived the storm. At times we will fall short, but it doesn't mean that what we have to give isn't worthy.

The culture does not hand belief-in-self out to women as a birthright the way it does to men. Instead, self-doubt seems to be our birthright. Self-doubt is part of being human, but it's often out of balance in women, affecting our ability to fully embrace the Upgrade. The idea of having wisdom is in competition with self-doubt, and it stops us from passing the baton to others.

I struggle with self-doubt too. Part of the process of writing this book is embracing the reality that I have a lot of knowledge about the female brain and about the life cycle of women. But I also personally have trouble with the idea of growing into a woman who has wisdom that is worthy of transmission. Writing this book means that I am watering that seed in myself and passing along my confidence that you have it too.

Fork in the Road: Upgrade or Downgrade?

At the very moment we have the chance to grow into a new emotional reality, our physical reality changes dramatically; some of those changes may provoke the brain to go into grief, shock, and denial. How we deal with our new realities determines whether we enter an Upgrade or a downgrade.

The first new reality is that your metabolism will slow to a crawl. Testosterone helps drive metabolism in the muscles; that in turn helps us burn more calories and have stronger muscle fibers. And now that all your hormone levels have dropped, including testosterone, it's easy to gain fat and lose muscle, making fat harder to lose. If you have a high school reunion or wedding coming up, it's not a three-week or three-month job to whack off five or ten pounds. It can take six months to a year to really make a difference. For many, it will mean almost no carbs, almost no alcohol, almost no processed food. Just veggies and lean protein, a teeny tiny bit of healthy fats, combined with weight-bearing and aerobic exercise four times a week. Even then, many of us will carry an extra five to ten pounds no matter how hard we try. Personally, I choose slightly looser-fitting clothes over going to war with my body's new metabolism.

Accepting the Challenge

Not stepping into the new reality and the new role of wisdom in the Upgrade might have long-term consequences for our cognitive health. Let me give you two solid reasons for stepping into an optimized Upgrade.

We have long known that when we actively engage in tasks and accomplish them, the reward system of the brain kicks in and releases dopamine. It's the feel-good chemical that floods our system during orgasm, a deep and satisfying conversation, or exercising to exhilaration. But what we didn't know, until research at the University of Washington School of Medicine revealed it, is the role certain cells in the brain play in suppressing dopamine when we give up. When we give in to self-doubt or even a bit of laziness and decide not to accomplish a goal, cells in the brain spring into action and block the reward system from activating. The more we let go of persistence and the more we drop off from follow-through, the stronger these dopamine-suppression circuits become. That change in brain activity toward demotivation presents a huge risk for depression. I am not talking about garden-variety sadness. I'm talking about can't-get-out-of-bed, don't-want-to-take-the-day's-next-step, completely debilitating, shades–closed–until–4:00 P.M. paralysis. Depression poses health risks as it causes us to drop self-care: heart disease, insomnia, dental decay, addiction, inflammation that can cause joint, artery, and cognitive damage. We become isolated as we continually cancel plans, depriving the brain of the essential vitamins it gets from connecting with others. We lose years of longevity as we let meaning and purpose slip away. When we decide not to activate our Upgrade, when we choose not to water our seeds of wisdom, we put everything we've spent a lifetime building at risk. And chances are we could be knocking ten years off our life span.

One way to snap yourself out of the brain's "I give up" circuits is to pull yourself into problem-solving mode. Plan an exercise schedule for a week, like a brief daily walk. Reengage with friends and/or family. In Pauline's case, I asked her to find ways to keep the dialogue open with her granddaughter, perhaps going to Los Angeles to help her get settled in her new apartment. Think about travel, learning something new, going to church, reading and finishing a book, calling one person every day.

The second reason for stepping into the Upgrade, for not giving up on our own wisdom, our own bodies, on our own health, is for others. Regardless of our self-doubt, it looks like the world could use our help. Not that we have to solve every major global problem—that would be impossible. But what we do in our daily interactions makes a difference. How we relate to others contributes either to peace or to conflict. It's up to us how we want to participate.

This is the opposite of "senioritis," those final days of high school or college when the grades are already in and your destiny is set, when you don't feel like going to class and you do the bare minimum to get by. Instead, ask yourself what else you want to do. Pull back to the thirty-thousand-foot view and notice what you might not have seen while still in the weeds of caretaking or the roles we are trapped in by cultural bias. It's time for us to go on the road, at least internally, with the same excitement to explore that Kerouac and the Beat poets had as they shattered convention and sought new meaning and purpose. We can, as they did, see ourselves and the world through new eyes, even if we need reading glasses to bring the details into focus.

Talking with Ceci, it was clear that her life had completely shifted. "The truth is," she said, "I'm feeling better than I ever have. I'm taking barre classes three times a week and a restorative yoga class once a week. I try to take some long walks in between. The best thing about that is I can sleep through the night and I can cough or sneeze without peeing!" I was really interested in Ceci's news. Many women struggle with some form of incontinence, especially after childbirth or hysterectomy, but may not be aware that pelvic-floor therapy or exercise like Pilates and barre can strengthen the muscles enough to alleviate the issue.

I could see that Ceci was really taking the Upgrade seriously. It was a joy to hear. She couldn't stop talking about what she was noticing. "I'm really seeing now how much food impacts my body—joint pain, energy, everything," she told me. "I've pretty much stopped drinking wine. It wakes me up with hot flashes and my hands hurt the next day. It just isn't worth it anymore. And it isn't that my problems have all evaporated. At my age, there's a greater likelihood that I will lose more friends, get sick, have more really big, really bad things happen. There's nothing I can do about it. There's no way to control anything in life. "

There is a lie about every decade that hides the truth about life's suffering. We tell those in their midtwenties that it's the time of their life, that they are hitting their stride, when those same young women are probably suffering their quarter-life crises and feel like they've been fourteen for ten years. We tell them that they'll calm down in their thirties, but then anxiety over marriage and kids—whether or not we have them—takes over our lives. We say that life begins at forty, but that's exactly when the Transition starts and can mean we take a wrecking ball to our relationships and career. The zero-Fs-given fifties are fabulous, and just when you feel great, you reach that phase when back-to-back catastrophes of losing friends and family and career become expected events. We don't know when catastrophe is going to hit, but we know it *is* going to hit. As long as we are alive, we will experience joy and suffering. But with every obstacle, we find the courage to keep going. We engage the problem solving of the prefrontal cortex, we keep moving physically to help the hippocampus find the energy to store new memories, and we spring to excitement as cortisol, particularly for women in the Upgrade, boosts our interest in learning new things.

The biggest benefit to having gone through those moments that bring us to our knees is learning the lesson of setting aside pride. We know what we don't know, and when you can't figure things out, as Mr. Rogers said, we find the helpers.

The Upgrade Circle

When you surround yourself with those who do what you want to be doing and are who you want to be, then that's what you preoccupy yourself with and that's what you become. Neurons that fire together wire together. If you are problem solving and seeing ahead, you are engaging circuits that get lost without use.

What you spend time pondering, that's what you become. The thought or emotion takes over your mind, and soon it impacts your behavior. Too many women get stuck in a phase I call Transition-mind. It's a necessary developmental stage that comes with the Transition. It is dominated by grief over what's been lost and confusion about what's to come. Many women cope by clinging to their before-the-Transition identity, dressing like teenagers and in some cases even dying on the operating table during a cosmetic procedure.

As little girls, teenagers, and young women, it was easier to shift out of transitions—there were clear cultural models for what we might look like in the next phase of life. But the Upgrade isn't yet visible. We've seen the cat-lady downgrade; that's not a place we are longing to go and it's not our only option.

I invite you to consider that even if you are done working, you are not done growing. Take time to really think about how you want to live this part of your life. Take a postretirement sabbatical if you need to, as I did. Listen to your body instead of overriding it. Spend some time becoming familiar with who you are at this point. Your brain may be hungry to learn new things. There are options other than volunteering or taking a job for much less money than a retired man would make. Choose what reignites your passion. I am challenging you to press forward in the cone of growth and fearlessly make yourself, your femaleness, visible. Repeat: You're not done yet. Choose the way you want to move through these years, and build the life of which you have just begun to dream.

The Neuroscience
of Self-Care

Chapter 6

Before the Transition, my massage therapist used to call me her Maserati; like the finicky sports car, I was always in the shop. I pushed myself to the limit and called on her when I blew past it, which was often. I muscled through everything, regardless of my body's signals of fatigue, illness, or pain. When I felt sick, I reached for something to suppress the aches caused by the storm of proteins called cytokines released by the immune system to attack an invading virus or bacteria. I learned to take Tylenol (acetaminophen) for those aches instead of Advil (ibuprofen); Advil kills antibodies and cytokines (and your stomach), which you need so that the immune system can do its job of killing hostile invaders like viruses and bacteria. You can bet I wrote myself a prescription for Tamiflu at the first sign of a virus, so that I wouldn't miss a beat at work.

For a while after I quit my job to help my husband recover from a surgery, I didn't change my habits. But I woke up one day in my early sixties with that familiar achy, fluish feeling and found myself doing something different. Instead of reaching for my prescription pad, I decided to rest and to trust my body, to respect the healing process and embrace feeling ill. I decided for the first time in my life to get out of the way and let my body use its natural powers. Respecting the wisdom of the body is huge for a doctor, especially when we can pretty much prescribe anything for ourselves except opioids or drugs like Valium. And for the first time, I didn't need to override symptoms and prop myself up to work.

Think about what it was like to be a newborn. Cycles of eating, sleeping, and getting rid of waste controlled not only your day but that of your caretaker. Every thought, plan, or movement was governed by the very strict schedule your tiny body needed. Meals, naps, and baths were all kept on a strict schedule, because neurohormones are stimulated by a regular light/dark cycle and a reliable routine lays the best foundation for brain development and overall health.

So let me ask you a question. When does the body stop needing a schedule? I didn't ask when we stop adhering to the body's schedule. That happens the minute we get woken up for school, still tired, not ready to be alert. Later we do it to ourselves, overriding the body's needs in order to get to an early meeting after being out or up too late the night before with kids, sick parents, friends, or a spouse.

The body we inhabit and the brain we count on never stopped being the baby that needs a schedule. Yes, your body had tons of resilience in your teens and twenties, but that was a temporary illusion, the last of it evaporating with the Transition. The stress buildup of being part of the sandwich generation, working and taking care of kids and aging parents, chips away at our physical health—sleeplessness, daytime agitation and anxiety, more colds and flus. As this wave gathers speed and size, you can bet it crashes right over the health of neurons, the brain cells we need for strong cognition.

When I was studying neurobiology at Berkeley, I was lucky enough to have neuroscientist Marian Diamond as my adviser. She was one of the main researchers to prove that as we age, brain-cell death is not inevitable, that we can indeed grow new neurons well into our eighties and nineties. She also let me in on another cool observation: that unlike what most of us thought, the brain's most important and populous cells are not neurons.

More than half of the brain is made of cells that clean up synaptic trash and bring nutrition to neurons, cells that can cause or reduce inflammation in the brain. Called microglia and astrocytes (or astroglia), until the late 1990s they were simply thought of as the mortar that held the brain together: "glia" is Greek for "glue." But they keep the neurons nourished and function as the gardeners and the Environmental Protection Agency of the brain. Sleep is the state in which they operate best.

Getting to sleep and staying asleep requires the balancing of a complex system of neurochemical waves rising and falling, hormones released and withdrawn that drive behavior. At least fifteen brain regions are involved in modulating the sleep/wake cycle, and neuroscientists still don't know how they all interact. But we do know something about what influences a proper cascade: sunlight, movement, food, beverages, and feelings of safety. Sleep is key to the unfolding of the Upgrade. If we don't get enough, we won't feel like exercising. If we don't exercise, the ability to think clearly diminishes, and it impacts our decision making on everything from food to relationships. We can initiate a virtuous cognitive cycle or a vicious cognitive cycle, depending on our actions and priorities.

Throughout the day, the brain is busy solving problems, creating new memories and new connections. The waste by-products of those synaptic firings are discarded proteins and molecules that need to be carted off before they rot or clump together in tangles that can spread through the brain, causing all kinds of cognitive trouble. The lymphatic system in the brain, the glymphatic system, is a system of rivers and streams of cerebrospinal fluid that run around neurons and synapses. When you're awake, the cells puff into that place, slowing down the flow of fluid. When you sleep, they retract, so that the rivers can swell and flush all the wasted proteins out, sending them off to the body's lymphatic system for filtering to the liver, which converts waste into forms the kidneys and bowel can expel. If that flushing in the brain doesn't happen, a buildup of sticky, toxic proteins gets in the way of synapses firing. If you've ever experienced brain glitches after a night of no sleep, sticky, toxic proteins left behind could be the cause.

With at least six uninterrupted hours of healthy, natural sleep, the brain's immune cells, microglia, have the chance to emerge like careful nighttime gardeners to trim away the overgrowth and carry out trash like extra tau and amyloid protein, while astrocytes restore and nourish neurons, rejuvenating their ability to communicate with one another. Astrocytes also form the brain's protective barrier, keeping toxins out, sorting for proper brain nutrients, and delivering those nutrients to neurons, like a mama bird finding food to bring to her babies. Keeping the brain clean and well fed, astrocytes and microglia are crucial to brain and cognitive health. Without restful sleep, they can't do their job of balancing debris and inflammation, and that can lead to the emergence of zombie cells.

The Dementors in the Harry Potter series have a special quality in their ability to drain happiness and hope from anyone to whom they come near. They are given one job in the books: to guard the prison of Azkaban. They are effective because proximity dampens the will of the prisoners to be free and the vitality needed to plan escape. In a state of inflammation, whether from lack of sleep or a proinflammatory lifestyle, the body has the capacity to create cells that act just like Dementors; cells that have stopped dividing and exist in a half-dead-half-alive state, like zombies, spewing toxic substances. Zombie cells are the primary drivers of toxic inflammation in the brain, especially the hypothalamus. When chronic inflammation happens in the brain, microglia and astrocytes are especially prone to going into zombie mode. Once that happens, those cells cease to clean out brain garbage. Instead, they generate new toxins that create even more inflammation, setting the stage for brain degeneration, faulty connections, and finally severe cognitive decline.

There may be hope in dealing with zombie cells. Studies in mice are showing that even when things in the brain look bad because of disease, destroying zombie cells helps restore the ability to retain newly formed memories. In the experiment, once the zombie cells were destroyed, signs of toxic inflammation were eliminated, there was no brain shrinkage, and there were no physical signs of cognitive impairment in the brain. Newer experiments in mice are indicating that flipping a genetic switch on astrocytes might turn them into neurons, i.e., make new brain cells. Drugs that mop up wasted brain proteins and zombie cells are being tried in humans now. For all of us and especially anyone suffering from brain degeneration, this line of inquiry could be promising.

Permission to Sleep

"I had never been a good sleeper," Chittra told me over her cup of herbal tea, "but at least I used to be able to get six straight hours." She looked exhausted and desperate; for three years, she had been unable to sleep more than a few hours. "I fall asleep easily. By ten thirty or eleven P.M. I am out cold. But I wake up at two A.M., and if I'm lucky I'll get another hour between six and seven A.M. I feel like I'm losing my mind. I now have a hair-trigger temper, I'm incredibly emotional, and my window for being able to work efficiently and think clearly during the day is very small."

Chittra had tried sleeping pills but concluded that they didn't help. While they may make you sleep, they don't actually improve sleep quality. Drugs interrupt our natural cycles of light sleep, deep sleep, and rapid eye movement (REM) sleep, during which we dream about what we've learned, giving the nervous system and brain a chance to rehearse and integrate new knowledge and information. The side effects of poor-quality sleep—irritability, moodiness, foggy thinking—are pretty much the same as those of insomnia, with the added obstacle of potential drug addiction. Long-term insomnia and use of sleeping pills are both associated with cognitive decline.

"So what are you doing now? Did you find any other sleep solutions?" I was fishing to see if Chittra had gone to common over-the-counter sleep remedies.

"Yes, I did find something that helped. A friend used Benadryl on her kids to get them to sleep on an overnight flight." She paused when she saw the look of horror on my face. "I know it's a last resort and it shouldn't be done," she interjected, "but I figured it wouldn't hurt me as an adult."

That's where Chittra was dead wrong. I wasn't all that upset about the impact of Benadryl on a child's brain. I was worried about Chittra's Upgrade.

Acetylcholine is a neurotransmitter with many roles in the nervous system and brain. It is a chemical messenger that activates muscles, makes us alert and able to learn new things, and plays a strong part in the formation and retention of memory. Healthy rising and falling of acetylcholine during waking and sleep cycles is essential to memory function. During waking hours, when acetylcholine is high, what we experience and learn during the day goes through a kind of first-draft wiring into the brain. During sleep, those memories undergo a reorganization process called memory consolidation, so that when we wake up in the morning, we remember not only what happened the day before but also what we need to do in the present. Consolidation requires us to practice in order to improve something we are working on learning and helps us remember what happened thirty years ago, in case any of it is relevant now. REM sleep, crucial to memory consolidation, changes in the second half of life. As women age, their nighttime sleep can be less steady because of drops in estrogen and hot flashes, among other things. Microawakenings become more common due to destabilized levels of melatonin, the neurohormone that helps us fall asleep and stay asleep. Sleep apnea becomes more common. All of this awakening contributes to problems with short-term memory.

Benadryl (diphenhydramine), like Tylenol PM, Nytol, Unisom, drugs to help with incontinence, tricyclic antidepressants like nortriptyline, and many other medications in this class, also share an additional property, what we call anticholinergic—the chemicals in these medications block acetylcholine, destroying the brain's ability to lay down memory pathways. Over time the suppression of acetylcholine can cause memory glitches and can block those muscles that release your poo and pee, making it harder to defecate or urinate. And acetylcholine blockage can also cause cognitive difficulties. The cognitive outcomes reported include mild cognitive impairment, confusion, forgetfulness, dizziness, falls, delirium, and decreased psychomotor speed and executive function. I've had patients come in looking like they are in the throes of dementia, when many times they've been taking too many anticholinergic drugs. If I catch it in time, getting patients off the medicine usually restores memory and mental clarity, not to mention bowel and bladder function. It turned out Chittra had sleep apnea.

Cortisol, Sleep, and Memory

Memory consolidation in sleep also requires low cortisol levels, especially during those first couple of hours of sleep. Cortisol is that hormone produced by the adrenals in a regular daily wave: high in the morning and low at night but also when the brain and nervous system get ready to respond to threat. So if you've had a fight or watched the news or read about violence right before sleeping, your brain will have a harder time with memory function from the cortisol alone. Chronic stress means chronic elevation of cortisol, making it nearly impossible to form new accurate memories during periods of extended grief and trauma.

A bit of neuroscience trivia dropped in my lap by Professor Diamond stuck with me over the years. When Albert Einstein passed away, he donated his brain to be studied. Its size and shape were unremarkable. But his astrocyte count was off the charts. He was famous for sleeping ten hours a night and taking a nap almost every day. A short nap, that is. If you sleep too long during the day, it will interrupt the nighttime cycle.

Einstein's high astrocyte count meant he had a clean and well-nourished brain. His habit of ten hours of sleep and regular, brief naps offers a lesson for the Upgrade. I know what it feels like when I've slept well: I am alert and energetic, the little things don't bother me as much, and I suddenly feel like my brain got a massive broadband upgrade. But making the time to get enough sleep may feel impossible or even counterintuitive. If you've had children and you work, you've spent most of your life sleep-deprived. Add to that the caretaking of aging parents, and it seems like all bets are off. As clarity fades from the morning jolt of caffeine and a stressed-out, foggy brain takes over, it makes getting through the day feel like a Herculean effort. Over time, it just feels true that life is exhausting.

Research is showing that as we head into our sixties, we need between seven and nine hours a night for the Upgrade to unfold. Less than six hours is associated with sterile inflammation, the kind of inflammation not caused by an infection. Yet insomnia is just about the most common complaint in adults sixty-five and older. But sleep problems are not inevitable, and usually they are not permanent. We can take simple actions during the day to prevent them. Here's Louann's Daily Sleep Plan, step one in activating the neuroscience of self-care:

- **Get direct sunlight.** Spend at least ten minutes in the sun on a sunny day, forty minutes on a cloudy day or use a light box. A thirty-minute walk first thing in the morning usually takes care of it.
- **Exercise to the edge of feeling tired.** Do something vigorous for thirty minutes before 3:00 P.M. If you do it later than that, chances are you will still have cortisol levels at bedtime that will interfere with sleep.
- **Limit caffeine.** Drink no more than one cup of something caffeinated, and only in the morning; for the best results, cut out caffeine altogether if you can.
- **Consume no stimulating substances in the afternoon.** Skip foods and drinks like dark chocolate and caffeinated sodas (which you should skip forever anyway).
- **Drink no alcohol in the evening or with dinner.** Alcohol may make you fall asleep faster, but it will likely cause you to wake up in the middle of the night.
- **Focus on protein and nonstarchy vegetables in the evening.** Carbs produce sugar, which creates short-term bursts of energy that raise cortisol.
- **Try to finish dinner by 6:00 p.m.**
- **Go to bed at the same time every night.** Schedule your wind-down and bedtime routine.
- **Get up one hour earlier if you've been feeling down.** This act alone cuts depression by a double-digit percentage. It means you have to go to sleep one hour earlier as well.
- **Shut off screens and devices at least thirty minutes before bedtime.**

- **Emphasize foods with L-tryptophan in the evening.** This is nature's sleep amino acid. You can find it in turkey, milk, cottage cheese, chicken, eggs, fish, pumpkin and sesame seeds, tofu, even bananas, but I'd eat those sparingly because of the high sugar load.
- **Nap sparingly, so as not to interrupt your nighttime sleep cycle.** Limit naps to ten to twenty minutes.
- **Invest in blackout shades and make sure the bedroom is quiet.** Or at least use an eyeshade and earplugs. Yes, you can get used to them. (I use custom-molded earplugs, since we live on a busy street.)
- **Make it cold.** Air temperature during sleep should be between sixty-six and sixty-eight degrees Fahrenheit. That doesn't mean you can't keep warm with blankets, and if your spouse complains, tell him to man up and get a heating pad. The super cold room temperature is good for him too.
- **If you get less than six straight hours of sleep, take a timed twenty-minute nap before 4:00 P.M.** Some who suffer chronic insomnia have been able to use three timed ten-minute naps per day to begin to downregulate the nervous system, aiding nighttime sleep. Long naps will absolutely interrupt nighttime sleep, so make your naps snack-length.

The Transition and Sleep

For me the Transition was a debilitating time. I woke up four or five times every night, the sheets soaked. I was going through two or three sets of pajamas nightly, and my days were miserable. Following the plan, I did start to sleep. My colleague Lynn, who was a few years younger and clearly going through the Transition, was showing signs of the irritability and memory glitches that come from insomnia. When I asked, she said she was doing just fine with sleep. Knowing women tend to be stoic, I probed a bit more.

"Are you really sleeping straight through the night? No little episodes of waking? No getting up to pee?" I asked.

"Ever since I did pelvic-floor therapy and have kept up with barre classes, nope, not waking up to pee anymore," Lynn said.

"No hot flashes? No warmth at night?" I pushed a little more.

"Well, I don't sweat or anything like you do, but three or four times a night I wake up hot and throw the blankets off. My husband usually covers me back up when he sees I'm getting cold," she admitted.

Waking up a little warm, rolling over, and falling back to sleep is fine if that happens once a night. But more than that and your restorative sleep is wrecked. Lynn's battle with the blankets was enough to keep her brain from getting the benefits of restorative sleep. I had a hunch a little adjustment to her HT would make the difference. I asked her to show me her compounding pharmacy prescription. As I suspected, her combination of estrogen, DHEA, and progesterone were bundled into one topical dose at night. For some people this works fine, but for many, the behaviors that these three hormones elicit from the brain can come into conflict. Estrogen and DHEA are a bit activating. They are great for getting the engine started and firing up the brain's cognitive powers. Perfectly suited to morning. But progesterone is the comfy, cozy hormone of self-care. Remember, progesterone increases the activity of the calming, Valium-like GABA system in the brain, relaxing us and making us sleepy. It's a robust behavior provocation that will demand actions like cuddling in a warm blanket near a fire with the best hot chocolate in the world during a cold winter rain. Self-nurturing is just what the body needs to settle in before sleep.

Estrogen stimulates the growth of new connections in the brain; it's like ultrafertilizer causing branches to grow everywhere. Before the Transition, in the second half of a cycle, progesterone comes in and down-regulates that overgrowth. Estrogen spikes during the Transition will cause much more overgrowth. On a microgram scale from ten to four hundred, estrogen can plummet to ten and spike to four hundred in the same day. The overgrowth can feel scrambling and disorienting and cause a lot of unfocused energy. Progesterone can be good for downregulating for better sleep and pruning the brain's overgrowth. But if you hit your brain with progesterone in the morning, it may make getting the day going a struggle.

Lynn was used to trying out new things, and she switched to using her progesterone at night. "I am sleeping like a baby," Lynn told me after three weeks. "I sleep straight through, no hot flashes, no waking up. I do wake up a little groggy some days and need to exercise and use the estrogen and DHEA right away."

"Great. Did you have to play with the dose at all?" I asked, because Lynn got her topical cream in syringes so that she could adjust the dose within a prescribed range. She's pretty sensitive and her doctor knows that. "I did," she said. "I ended up cutting everything in half. My doctor was upping estrogen to take care of hot flashes. It turned out that the higher dose wasn't making the hot flashes better, and I was getting really edgy. Once I found the right dose for me, I started to settle into a really comfortable sleep rhythm."

Estrogen plus DHEA can push us to the razor's edge of vigilance. If you have that wound-up feeling that doesn't go away no matter how much yoga you do, consider taking progesterone at bedtime. If you do, add it in tiny doses, upping it slowly over time, giving your brain and nervous system the time they will need to adjust and consider stopping DHEA. The same should be done with any hormone. Add it slowly, increasing in tiny increments if you are sensitive like Lynn. Most ob-gyns won't know to do this. Remember, their training is for handling high-risk pregnancies and cancer surgery. Neurologists won't know either. They are trained for treating MS, Parkinson's, strokes, Alzheimer's, and others. None of them are trained in how our hormones impact the brain. Endocrinologists are trained but generally don't practice in this area. If you can find one with experience outside thyroid, diabetes, and rare endocrine issues like the disease of the adrenals, Addison's, and Cushing's, you're lucky. Although as a psychiatrist I was trained to understand the hormone as a neurochemical, I hadn't been trained in the specific issues of women until I got interested in them myself. There is no medical subspecialty that particularly trains in HT for women, so don't expect your doctor to know. Ob-gyns, family physicians, functional medicine doctors, and nurse practitioners who prescribe hormones will know the most. Whoever you work with, you'll likely have to teach them how to treat you. That idea doesn't go over well with many doctors, so keep searching until you find a medical *partner*.

The thing to remember about hormones is that even if they are making you feel good, more is not always better. There is a sweet spot that will work best for you. It will be different from someone else's, and it may be different from a so-called normal range reported by a lab. You'll know what's normal for you because you will sleep, you will not have hot flashes, and you will feel better.

Reducing Stress

Chronic sterile—not caused by an infection—inflammation from the body's stress and threat system might be the single biggest long-term threat to healthy cognition in the Upgrade. By now you know the cascade of problems from chronic cortisol release, especially the risk of intractable melancholy. And it doesn't take a brain scientist to tell you that stress can make it hard to sleep. But the body's nervous system offers plenty of inflection points for teaching it to stand down from red alert.

Even before her Transition, Diane, now sixty, admits to having had a fairly explosive personality, triggered easily by insecurity and fear. "My sense of self got tugged at daily during what you call the fertile phase," she said in a conversation about her journey to self-care. "It was hard to stay strong when the men around me seemed to be working overtime to prove I wasn't good enough, or to shut me out of opportunities." I knew what she meant. It happened to me all through med school and in several early jobs. "It got harder to handle as soon as I hit the Transition. I kept getting knocked over by things that hadn't bothered me in a long time. Sleep was harder. Internally I felt like I was completely out of control.

The confidence and certainty that had sustained me earlier in my life just vanished."

I asked Diane how she started to find her balance. "When I was a kid," she said, "I was a pretty serious musician. I played the oboe; I competed and performed a lot. If you get too nervous, your hands get cold and you lose the fine control you need over your fingers. Anxiety makes it harder to control the tiny muscles in the face and around the mouth that you need to recruit in order to produce a steady sound. And if you can't calm down, the stomach tightens, keeping you from getting a deep enough breath to play through a phrase." Everything Diane was telling me was an indication of the sympathetic stress reaction takeover.

"So what helped?" I asked.

"They taught us alternate-nostril breathing. When my mind started feeling scrambled during the Transition, somehow I remembered this technique. I did alternate-nostril breathing while waiting for my toast or the Nespresso machine to finish, any opportunity, until it became a habit during stressful moments. It led me to yoga and meditation, which have given me more targeted and sophisticated tactics to keep the threat system in my brain from overwhelming my body."

Diane had something there; alternate-nostril breathing is an ancient technique that can trick the vagus nerve into activating the body's calming circuits. Try it sometime. In a moment of activation, plug your right nostril and take a fine, slow breath through your left nostril. Then plug your left nostril and breathe out a fine, slow breath through the right. Try to keep the breath from being audible, even to yourself. It can help to imagine breathing in and out through a pinhole. Do that three times— plug the right on the inhale, plug the left on the exhale—and then switch, plugging the left on the inhale, the right on the exhale for three rounds. The final three breaths should be fine, slow inhales and exhales through both nostrils. (For more on this technique, see appendix, page 258.)

There are nine breaths in one round of this practice, and here's how it works on the brain. Inside your nostrils are tiny little hairs that have nerves at their roots. Their job is to communicate changes within the sinus passages to the brain. Those little hairs expect that when you breathe in, the nerves in both nostrils will be stimulated. When we disrupt that expectation by closing one nostril, it alerts the brain to pay attention to the breath. The cerebellum registers that balance is off and recruits a keen, settled attentiveness. Following a predictable pattern engages the cortex, the thinking organ of the brain, to connect with that little bit of alertness that has been provoked. I use this technique throughout the day to settle triggered brain circuits. It allows the nervous system to get out of threat-response mode, and anything I can do to get myself out of distress supports cognitive function both short term and long term.

In the Upgrade, we can consciously activate healthy circuits for social connection, safety, and self-nurturing. Visualization is one of the most powerful ways for this to occur. At Emory University's Compassion Center, they have studied the effects of meditative engagement with what they call a *nurturing moment*. As participants are asked to recall or imagine a moment of protection, safety, peace, or nurturing, whether spiritual, among other people, or in nature, what surprises people the most is that all the circuitry that has experienced caring, whether giving or receiving, can be activated easily. It takes just a bit of concentration on the details of an experience or imagined moment of safety or protection, calm or refuge, to reawaken it as though it were happening in the present moment. Whether we've had good or bad parenting, good or bad marriages, the fact that we are alive today means that at some point someone cared unconditionally for us, even if it was just for one moment. I know I have a nurturing-moment memory of sitting on my father's lap while we were reading a big animal book and my mother was beaming while taking a photo of us. Rehearsing these moments to the point that we feel the presence of their impact means that in tough moments we are more likely to find ways to reconnect, to activate the bonds of the Upgrade. I use mine every morning as part of my prayer and meditation practice (see appendix, page 253). It's the first step in a compassion training protocol. And just so you know, the entire protocol has been proven to have a greater impact on helping the brain and body recover more quickly from stress and reducing inflammation than simple mindfulness of the present moment or even support groups. I now teach this to my patients.

The Gut Brain

What and when we eat has almost as big an impact on mood and cognition as do sleep and stress. And it's all because every single body has two brains. And no, it's not what you think. I'm talking about the one that stretches from your esophagus to your anus: the gastrointestinal tract.

Terri had been waking up every morning at 5:00 A.M. in a cold sweat, heart pounding, her insides in turmoil, feeling terrified. She called me because her GP had diagnosed these episodes as panic disorder and wanted her to start on antianxiety meds. Terri was concerned about taking them; her sister had had a bad reaction to a similar drug, and her experience of getting off it had taken her to a psychologically frightening brink. Having known Terri for so many years, and having treated so many patients with panic disorder, my instincts told me that this wasn't panic. So I asked her to try an experiment. "Get your doctor to write a prescription for five tablets of five milligrams of Valium," I suggested. "And then do the following: When you have one of these episodes, break one of the pills into quarters. Put one quarter under your tongue and let it dissolve." When Valium is dissolved under the tongue, it gets the chemicals into the bloodstream and to the brain more quickly; Terri would feel the effect of it within a few minutes, rather than waiting the twenty or more it could take to absorb into the bloodstream through her digestive tract.

An overactive amygdala is a key brain organ that triggers that heart-racing, out-of-body, sweaty feeling of impending doom. If Terri was having a panic attack, then Valium, which quiets the amygdala's fear circuits, should make both the symptoms and the panic lessen or even disappear. But if it wasn't a panic attack, then while the fear might subside, the symptoms would remain. And that would mean something else was causing Terri's attacks.

In Terri's case, it was not panic. "Louann, I did what you suggested for a week," she told me, "and every single time, the fear went away but the intestinal turmoil, cold sweat, and heart pounding didn't stop." My hunch was right. Terri's emotional overwhelm was coming from another part of her body, a part whose language is vague yet powerful in the control it exerts over the brain and nervous system.

Further testing showed that Terri had severe, undiagnosed food allergies. I can already hear the question bubbling up, because I once asked the same one: How does an allergy that's not life-threatening, an allergy that's not causing your throat to close (anaphylaxis), cause a feeling of panic?

An allergy happens when ingestion of a normally benign substance, like pollen, peanuts, gluten, or soy, provokes an immune response from the body, which attacks the substance as though it were a dangerous invader that needed to be annihilated. Allergens leave traces along the various filtration layers of the digestive tract. The immune system, a huge proportion of which is in the GI tract, attacks whatever tissue these traces attach to, causing inflammatory reactions—just as a wound turns red and swells.

The entire gastrointestinal tract, from your esophagus to your anus, is wrapped in a web of interconnected neurons burrowed within the bowel wall that regulates motility and secretions. It has 50 to 100 billion neurons, the same number of neurons as in the entire spinal cord. It's the GI tract's very own nervous system, which regulates the key functions of the bowel: movement of food and nutrients, secretion and absorption of fluid, repair of the bowel lining, and blood flow through it. Called the ENS (enteric nervous system), it's such a huge number of neurons that it's called the body's second brain. The ENS can signal the brain via the vagus nerve about what's going on in the GI tract, especially if there is distress, as in an allergic response, and try to get the conscious mind to form an idea for corrective action. That's the usual mechanism for the nerve/brain dance. It works great when signals take the form of a clear message to the conscious mind: *Ouch, the stove is hot. Move your hand.* Or if you just ate something rotten: *Throw up now.* But when the signal is less clear and travels up a long nerve like the vagus that attaches to and communicates with the parts of the brain that control unconscious functions, those signals can be more subtle and harder to register.

The Vague Signals of the Vagus Nerve

Widely distributed through the voice box, chest, and gut, the vagus nerve—"vagus" comes from the same Latin root as "vagabond"—is a long and wandering nerve. It attaches at the brain stem—the part of the brain that is in charge of functions like breathing, heart rate, blood pressure, body temperature, wake and sleep cycles, emotional well-being, digestion, sneezing, coughing, vomiting, and swallowing. It is partly responsible for balancing both our threat response (sympathetic nervous system) and our calming response (parasympathetic nervous system). Without the potential calming effect, sensations like tightness or uneasiness in the stomach and throat that can be a precursor to fear; a burning in the throat, chest, or upper belly that can come just before an explosion of anger; or a lump in the throat that is a harbinger of sadness can make the difference between being able to wait out a feeling and having an emotional explosion. It's often called the sixth sense because of how sensitive it is, and it also connects the brain to the gut.

The inside of the intestines is also populated by a vast jungle of single-celled creatures that help us process what enters the body and bloodstream, extracting nutrients and expelling waste. The usually healthy bacteria that take up residence in our intestines help us grow, develop, and live a healthy life. The flora and fauna in our intestines—collectively known as the microbiome—are essential to helping our immune system do its job of maintaining balance between inflammation—when confronted with an invader—and anti-inflammation (regulation when the threat is gone). We've known that for decades. But fascinating new research is indicating that the microbiome has several ways to impact the brain; it may strongly influence mood, clarity of thought, even emotions.

Through the ENS–vagus–brain stem circuit, the microbiome sends up *We're okay, so you're okay* or *We're not okay, so you're not okay* signals that are influenced by the environmental shifts caused by food, sleep, travel, and exercise habits. It makes you feel tired, moody, or even anxious when you switch up a diet or keep an irregular schedule. Think about the last time you spent a day or two not being able to eat properly. No energy? A little irritated? Cytokines, chemicals released from immune cells, can be responsible for that feeling of sickness—so lethargic you can't get out of bed, foggy-headed, fearful, down, or even depressed. As the insula scans to see if everything is okay, via the ENS–vagus–brain stem circuit, the microbiome might be complaining loudly if there are inflammatory cytokines because of an autoimmune response: *No! Not okay! A lot of inflammation in here. It's too hot and too acidy and we can't survive!*

At the same time, the language of the vagus—the nerve responsible for transmitting the microbiome's signals to the brain—is, well, vague. It has two extremes that issue clear commands: *Total well-being, so keep doing what you're doing* or *This is poison, so vomit now*. Everything in between is pretty unclear. When the microbiome is unhappy, the signal might be to eat more, sleep more, flop on the couch, cry, or panic.

Scientists in Canada proved the microbiome/anxiety connection in 2011 by transplanting poop from a group of mice genetically bred to be anxious into the intestines of a group that was not. After a short period of time, the nonanxious mice behaved like the anxious mice just from the change in their microbiome caused by the poop from the anxious mice. The opposite turned out also to be true: Transplanting poop from a healthy donor made the anxious mice calmer.

When the immune system goes into overdrive, as it did in Terri's case, and kicks up inflammation in the gut in response to allergens, the ENS will detect a threat and will set off any alarm it can. The lives of the microbiome are on the line, and they don't have a great translator in the vagus. As Terri's allergens caused a massive destabilization to the community of roughly 100 trillion bacteria communicating with her ENS, the poor little creatures were screaming for help, but because of the vagus, the message was arriving in an unrecognizable language.

Upgrading the Gut-Brain Team

It wasn't a surprise that Terri's symptoms were worsening during her Transition. Microbiome composition changes with age, influenced by the shift in hormone levels. Progesterone helps bolster the microbiome's population of lactobacillus, which is protective against depression and anxiety. Estrogen helps regulate the microbiome and maintain the diversity needed to keep it in balance. Lower estrogen means the body has a harder time adjusting to inflammation that can disturb the balance of bacteria. When that happens, it can kick off a hostile environment, allowing the growth of hostile bacteria that can eventually impact mood and cognition. When unfriendly bacteria start to outpace the supportive bifidobacterium and lactobacillus, particularly *Lactobacillus reuteri,* it not only impacts mood but also can interfere with memory. *L. reuteri,* which we receive from our mothers at birth, provides protection from unfriendly species. Its presence in human microbiomes decreases both with age and with overuse of antibiotics in childhood and beyond—antibiotics kill not only harmful bacteria but your friendly ones as well. Artificial sweeteners, including stevia, also cause microbiome imbalance and changes in the gut/brain signaling. Combine this with the effects of dwindling estrogen and progesterone, and the imbalance of bacteria not only exacerbates the brain fog and mood changes of the Transition but also can make Swiss cheese out of the digestive tract's lining. When that happens, toxins and bacteria can leak through tiny gaps into your body instead of being flushed out. When these foreign substances hang around where they aren't supposed to be, it triggers chronic inflammation, which in turn can start a cascade of issues that lead to cognitive decline. This is how inflammation in one part of the body can trigger inflammation in the brain; inflammation in the brain is a cause of cognitive decline.

New studies are showing that the microbiome can be a contributing factor in brain diseases like MS, stroke, Parkinson's, and Alzheimer's. In 2019 researchers at Johns Hopkins did an experiment with mice to explore the connection between the gut microbiome and brain health. In the experiment, the mice were given bacteria that would harm their gut and cause them to develop Parkinson's. Parkinson's is a disease that causes nerve cell damage and cell death which in turn causes the decrease in dopamine in the brain. Without dopamine, movement gets harder, everything from trying to put a spoon to one's mouth to swallowing. In the experiment, they separated the mice into two groups. In one, they simply observed the progression of the disease. In the other group, they cut the vagus nerve, interrupting the gut's messages to the brain. The group with the intact vagus nerve developed Parkinson's. The group with the severed nerve did not. They concluded that some injurious gut proteins created by the bacteria were signaling the brain via the vagus nerve and causing Parkinson's.

The same study also showed that we don't have to sever the vagus nerve to prevent the microbiome from sending unhealthy messages to the brain. We can take action through diet and exercise, both of which have a positive impact on microbiome health. The healthier the microbiome, the healthier the signals sent to the brain, and the better chance we have for optimizing cognition in the Upgrade. Everything that causes weight gain is also bad for the microbiome. (See appendix, page 268.) And what's bad for the microbiome is bad for cognition. This doesn't necessarily mean you should go out and start gobbling down a bunch of probiotics. What it does mean: Focus on foods high in fiber, which promotes regeneration that may help protect the brain from both Parkinson's and Alzheimer's diseases. And to grow and support the right kinds of helpful bacteria, follow the Mediterranean diet, with lean proteins, lots of leafy greens, and a small amount of healthy fats (see appendix, page 268). And timing is everything: Make sure you leave twelve to sixteen hours between dinner and breakfast. It stresses the metabolism in a good way, just like building muscles in the gym. Giving the GI tract a rest during these hours helps the microbiome flourish. And even without changing your diet, moderate aerobic exercise, thirty to sixty minutes three times a week, has been shown to increase the diversity of microbes in your gut and reduce intestinal inflammation in just six weeks, although scientists don't yet understand why.

Unless you have other medical conditions, a probiotic supplement can be helpful, especially after you've been given a course of antibiotics, which destroy the good, brain-supporting bacteria. The microbiome needs to be seeded and given good fertilizer to grow back healthy. If it's recommended that you take some, get a good concentrated probiotic supplement with 200 billion cells, and make sure it contains *L. reuteri*.

When the microbiome is populated by friendly flora, those bacteria trigger balance and well-being. You can eat and exercise your way to health, but you'll have to do it without the usual high-sugar and high-fat comfort foods or artificial sweeteners, which are the fastest route to a downgrade. There is a beautiful garden in our guts working to nourish our body, cognition, and mood, growing what we need to fuel the Upgrade. But it needs our support in order to do its job.

Food, Alcohol, and Cognition

I have been involved in Weight Watchers for twenty-five years. I am pretty compliant and I have the data to prove it, collected over the course of time. I don't drink much these days because it interrupts my sleep and I don't feel well afterward. But Sam and I were out at a friend's one night for dinner, and I decided I was going to join in on everyone's fun. The couple we were visiting are serious gourmets and have amazing knowledge of wine, so I had a little red and a second piece of the flourless chocolate torte they had made. It was delicious. All that sugar gets the brain very excited—glucose is its favorite fuel, easy to access and to use. So I was in a bubbly mood. We went home, I fell asleep quickly, and I was happy with my FOMO-driven splurge.

At 3:00 A.M., I woke up, heart pounding, drenched in sweat. I was scared and spent two hours thinking I was having a heart attack. At around five thirty I realized it was reflux, so I took an antacid and fell back to sleep around six. When I got out of bed at nine, I was groggy and my hands hurt. My fingers and knuckles were red and every joint ached.

Inflammation in the body is, at its best, a choreography of healing processes. We cut ourselves, and proinflammatory cytokines rush to the site to start building a bridge for healing. Similarly, we can trigger a wound response inside the body through the wrong food and drink, lack of sleep, or lack of exercise. Just a tad too much sugar can stimulate the release of those proinflammatory cytokines that cause redness and swelling, but this time inside the body. It happens more easily as we age; the body becomes more susceptible to inflammation.

In the brain, proinflammatory cytokines reduce the signaling in areas that stimulate muscles, causing that feeling of not wanting to move, suppressing motivation. Brain inflammation shuts down energy production in neurons, slowing cognitive processes including memory. In a state of inflammation it's harder to read, work, or concentrate for any length of time. When cytokines remain in an overactivated state, as they are in chronic inflammation, they can have significant impact on the female brain by disrupting sleep and decreasing the release of feel-good neurochemicals such as serotonin and dopamine. Instead of making the feel-good neurochemicals free-floating and available to the right circuits so that we will feel and sleep better, cytokines encourage the brain to suck them all back up. When that happens, you won't feel their benefit, the experience of well-being.

In one fell swoop, proinflammatory cytokines can cause moodiness, low libido, anxiety, insomnia, intractable melancholy, and muscle weakness. In a healthy homeostasis, the inflammatory process is a beautifully choreographed dance performed by the immune system, in which proinflammatory and anti-inflammatory cytokines are in balance. But things get tricky when cytokines linger too long, past their usefulness in repairing tissues. When we ingest a consistent flow of sugary food and drink, cytokines overstay their welcome and inflammation becomes chronic; the result is progressive tissue *damage* rather than repair.

The decrease in estrogen after the Transition makes it harder for the body to be resilient in the face of inflammation, and with weight gain around the middle, toxic belly fat also releases proinflammatory cytokines, which in turn sparks chronic low-grade inflammation. A 2013 study in Iowa even showed an association between inflammation and a shortened life span.

In amounts greater than one glass of wine, alcohol becomes an inflammatory brain toxin, damaging the ends of neurons and impairing the growth of new cells, especially in the hippocampus, the brain's organ of memory. Several brain imaging studies and tests for memory and learning skills show that excessive drinking increases the risk of cognitive decline and dementia, and some are pretty alarming. For instance, a 2013 study in Australia found that 78 percent of people diagnosed with alcohol-use disorder displayed some form of dementia or brain pathology. The effects of alcohol on the brain are so powerful that there are even specific types of dementia, distinct from Alzheimer's disease or vascular dementia, that are called "alcohol-related." Heavy alcohol use can literally restructure your brain, causing permanent damage, especially in the frontal cortex, which is your planning, judgment, and cognition center. Structural changes can be permanent.

The kicker: The bad effects of alcohol on an aging brain are more damaging in women than in men. The toxic effects can make the symptoms of the Transition worse, slowing metabolism and increasing the risk of osteoporosis and insomnia.

And if that weren't bad enough, women in their sixties today are drinking heavily more than ever, even more than men of the same age. Studies at the National Institutes of Health show that while men drink out of social pressure, women do so in response to emotional pain. Research on women and alcohol in the last twenty years has shown that damage to the brain, liver, and metabolism happens faster for us, even for those of similar muscle mass and weight to a man. Light alcohol use—no more than one drink per day for women—may actually be neuroprotective against dementia. But even one glass can exacerbate hot flashes and sleeplessness.

I know. It's not the best news, but we work with what we've got.

The combination of sugar and alcohol in the female brain can turn the Upgrade into a downgrade faster than you can uncork a bottle of champagne. In many post-Transition women, sugar and alcohol can trigger some concerning inflammatory consequences. Increases in inflammatory markers, which can be measured by your doctor, are a direct threat to the female brain and manifest themselves in both cognitive decline and intractable melancholy. A 2019 study showed that high levels of CRP (C-reactive protein, a common marker of inflammation) in older adults predicted worsening mood symptoms just twelve months after elevated levels were detected. And over time, that lack of positive mood also predicted increasing inflammation—a vicious cycle becomes established. In a French study of eighty-to-eighty-five-year-olds, those with the highest levels of IL-6, another cytokine marker of inflammation, showed the greatest shrinkage in their brains, which is a sign of predementia. Inflammation may be a powerful factor in brain shrinkage—and thus cognitive decline—as we age. And it's a powerful factor in chronic melancholy and insomnia.

On the flip side, food, sleep, and exercise can be medicine. Eating anti-inflammatory foods at the right times, keeping belly fat under control, and making sure you're moving enough can turn inflammation around, making a huge difference in mental sharpness now and for the future. We can eat, sleep, and exercise our way to an Upgrade.

———

I don't remember where this came from, but when I heard it, it stuck in my mind: "'Eat, pray, love' takes on another meaning at this time: I eat less, I pray more that it doesn't make me fat, and I try and fail every day at loving the body I have." Like most women in our culture, I've spent a lifetime denying myself food that I wanted in order to look a certain way. Now I've tried to flip that formula on its head and think about what's important to me in the Upgrade. Yes, I want to be healthy and look great, but my priority is having a strong, sharp, clear, and quick brain. That's the only way to have a second half that's even better than the first.

Keeping Your Reserve Tank Full

During the fertility era, what we prioritized was pretty much dictated by biology and fear. If you ask most women what they want more time for in the Upgrade, they say self-care, whether it's exercise, rest, or transformative spiritual practice. It's a wake-up call in the Transition. It announces itself with a feeling that you are burning too deeply into your reserves, that if you don't do something soon you'll be in serious trouble. I hear this from women as they enter the Transition all the time. We tend to ignore those signals until we break.

"I've been saying for years that I needed a break," said my colleague Lynn, "that I needed a vacation. And when I used to blow past something like that, I might get a cold or a flu that would put me in bed for a few days or a week. But this time I got a cold, the flu, and pneumonia, and I was out for two months. And recovery? They say six months before I can feel normal, two years before my lungs stop being triggered by irritants."

What I urge women to hear at this moment is one message: Trust your body, trust your brain, hear the cries of the nervous system. If you are alive in the second half, you came from people who genetically were tough. They were survivors. You made it to the second half because you have better-than-average genes. So even if they don't work the way they used to, recognize that you can trust your body and brain. But the approach has to be different.

You have to give the body the right conditions to heal. Rest, nutrition, sleep, exercise, daylight, managing your threat response, being silent to listen for what the body needs. Sometimes that will be cardio, sometimes restorative yoga. Listen to and trust what it says, and do your best not to override it with fear or anxiety over how long it's taking to get better. The time frame of healing changes in the Upgrade. It's messy. Things we thought we got over come and go and take their own time.

The Upgrade, if we listen, teaches us that if we want to keep our cognition, we have no option but to hew closely to what the brain and body need. And it's often not an option. When the burdens are too big, learn to unbite your tongue. Find a way to say, "It's your turn. My body needs to fall apart. Stop asking me for things. I need ten minutes. I need a day. Please figure it out yourself." We can begin to shift the environment around us so that it becomes more healing and supportive. We have the choice to recognize our responsibility for our decisions. We have the freedom now to change everything.

Your Brain in Search of Connection

Chapter 7

"I never imagined how in love I would fall," Sherry told me on our weekly call. Widowed for five years, she had sold her café in Connecticut and moved to Arizona to be near her son David's family. She has three grandchildren and a great relationship with her daughter-in-law, Elise. She's a big part of the children's lives, participating in their school activities and staying with them when Mom and Dad need a getaway. She's become a coconspirator to her sixteen-year-old granddaughter's fashion rebellions: If her mother won't let her have it, Grandma will get it for her—within reason, of course. All done with a wink and a nod to Elise. "That part of my life with the grandkids is great," the seventy-two-year-old tells me. "But don't kid yourself. It's hard and lonely. I am nowhere near my friends on the East Coast, and there's only so much David wants me around. With that move I went through a really big depression a couple of years ago. As you know, I didn't think I would ever climb out of it."

The part of the brain that registers social pain from isolation, the anterior cingulate cortex (ACC), is also part of our basic primate empathy circuit. They are the same circuits that help us figure out what to do when a baby cries or another's face expresses sadness. The ACC is part of what enables us to feel and react to another's emotions and pain. High levels of cortisol from feeling isolated can make that wiring go askew over time. We misread the cues of language and faces; we stop responding to sadness. If we remain isolated long enough, reconnecting won't feel like an option. The attempts of others to reach out to us will feel hostile. We are more likely to lash out and push family, friends, and qualified mental health practitioners away.

The phrase "I could die of loneliness" is not just a melodramatic cliché. It's both a deep evolutionary memory and a physical reality. Wired to live in the wilderness, human beings, like most other mammals, have the best chance of thriving in groups. When there are others to help share the load of gathering or cultivating food, of caring for one another, of fending off attackers, survival comes from collaboration. For women, this instinct is strong. For us, smaller and often with young children in tow, safety has always come in numbers, especially when faced with a violent male.

One of the jobs of the brain and its nervous system is to signal us to engage in acts that lead to survival. When we are thirsty, we feel dry, headachy, tired, and foggy. We hydrate and the nervous system stops sending hormones and chemicals to the brain that push us to drink. In time, symptoms go away. When we are hungry, the stomach tightens and growls, sometimes painfully; we feel exhausted, stressed, and moody. When we eat, the symptoms dissipate and the nervous system tells the brain that it is safe to close the refrigerator door and leave the kitchen.

Connecting with others—the need to belong—is as deep a survival instinct as eating, drinking, and sleeping. Social connection activates the brain's physical reward circuitry far more than researchers imagined. At the University of Chicago, they found that the brain's strong pleasure pathways related to social connection have evolved over hundreds of millions of years in response to the success of collaboration in survival. The joy of belonging brings an accompanying feeling of lightness and ease in the body. At the same time, they found that social pain piggybacks on the body's physical pain circuits. So when we are hurt or heartbroken or alone, that feeling can become actual pain. There is no louder signal to most nervous systems than a blow or cut to the body. It stops everything and lets us know that we are in danger. Researchers hypothesize that it's probably evolution—the deadly consequences of being alone in the wild or left unprotected as a helpless newborn—that made it possible for social pain to hijack physical pain circuits.

Belonging circuitry is among the strongest in any mammal. But recognizing the symptoms of lacking connection is much harder than recognizing the symptoms of hunger, thirst, or sleepiness. We can attribute lethargy to hunger, lack of sleep, or exertion. We can attribute body aches to the onset of flu, an allergy, arthritis, lack of sleep, or a life stress. But we rarely hear the nervous system's calls to solve isolation, drowned out as they are by a collective cultural boom box playing a rugged, individual-worshipping "survival of the fittest" anthem on full blast.

Let's just bust that lone-wolf lie here and now. No one does anything alone. It's neither theoretically nor logically possible. Without others you don't have life. Without others you have nothing to eat or drink, no home to live in, no roads to travel, no work, no source of income. Whether they intend to or not, the actions of others help us survive every moment we are alive.

Columbia University psychologist Scott Barry Kaufman analyzed the results of several studies on gender and personality conducted across various academic institutions. Using personality traits, he was able to determine whether a brain was female or male with 85 percent accuracy. So when we say that dominance, aggression, and rigid hierarchies are male personality traits, we can say, according to Kaufman's work, that the statement is true. The research shows just as reliably that women are more likely to be agreeable and men more likely to be disagreeable. How this plays out is that women tend to value collaboration, transparency, and fluid organizational structures, while men admire the lone wolf and value fixed hierarchies that stay in place for long periods of time.

So when we buy into the worship of self-sufficiency, we are mostly operating from an introjected male value. When we are sad and roll up like a potato bug, refusing to reach out for fear of being seen as weak, we are overriding the life-giving survival mechanism of connection. And we are endangering our health. Not just as women but as human beings.

The Tent of "Me"

It wasn't just the mere act of moving to a new city that was disorienting to Sherry. It was incredibly hard as her brain, her mirror neurons—those cells in the brain responsible for reflecting the nervous system of another, helping to create a bridge of empathy—and nervous system went through the adjustment of losing the former affirmations of her visceral sense of herself. It wasn't just the loss of the familiar friends; it was also the dry cleaner, the woman who did her hair, the clerks she saw at the grocery store, who in regular interactions shaped her sense of self. It would take years for the nervous system to adjust to the shift in feedback: both the loss of familiar human beings and the new input of those who were beginning to enter into her life.

Awareness of how the brain and nervous system incorporate others into our sense of self means we can collaborate with it instead of being at its mercy. We can Upgrade that sense of self into who we have always wanted to be.

When the brain constructs a sense of self, it must do so via the experience transmitted by the entire nervous system. An embodied sense of self is generated and contained as a unique combination of patterns across multiple neurons in each circuit that contributes to the construction. The feeling of "Me" is stored in patterns of nerve impulses across widely distributed systems, which interact not only with many complex circuits of the brain but with all the large and teeny tiny nerves in your skin, your organs, your blood vessels. Experience, encounters with others, and the imprints they leave on the nervous system are major components of our sense of what it feels like to be "Me" in my own skin. With every connection and bond, the nervous system matches and incorporates the expressed thoughts and unexpressed behavior patterns of those with whom we become familiar. The more frequently our nervous system comes into contact with another's nervous system, the more influenced our own becomes by theirs, the more we incorporate the feeling of being around them into the feeling of "Me."

While the brain's motivation and reward system, via the neurochemicals dopamine and oxytocin, is triggered intermittently by new people and new discoveries, it is turned on full blast and kept purring along through consistent contact with those to whom we feel closeness and love.

Sitting or walking or talking together, our heartbeats attune, our blood pressure syncs, and we begin to breathe in unison. Our nervous system triggers muscle movements in response to unnoticed cues; like musicians playing in an ensemble, we sense more than see what others need from us and find ourselves responding to subtle signals without conscious awareness. This attunement, when reciprocated, grows into attachment: the very deep sense that a partner, child, parent, or sibling is an integral part of who we are.

When they are not there, not only do we miss them, but we physically miss who we are when we are in their presence. Nerve signals that we rely on to tell us everything is okay with the "Me" that feels familiar become scrambled when those most familiar to us are no longer in our lives, just as they are scrambled when a body part is removed. If there is a dramatic or abrupt change in a relationship with someone to whom we are close, to whom we are used to being around, the brain and nervous system crave their proximity intensely. The nervous system goes into acute withdrawal with the death of or rupture with a spouse, child, parent, close family member, or old friend. Signals indicating lack of familiarity start setting off alarms that something isn't right. Grief can become complicated by the nervous system's distress, overwhelming us with anxiety, fear, and sleep interruption, as well as dramatic changes in appetite, food preference, and libido. It can feel extreme, like our world is coming to a catastrophic end.

Anticipation of the lack of social connection, when you feel you've been treated unfairly or you're afraid someone will be pissed over what you did or didn't do or said or didn't say, is among the most painful physical and emotional experiences we have. Women who divorce around the time of the Transition have told me this feeling is particularly strong as their married friends begin to drop them, in some cases because they had socialized as couples but in others because some married women are afraid a divorced woman will go after their partners. The pain circuits triggered by the feeling of being ostracized are very physical. It feels apocalyptic.

During the struggle of the Transition, as she focused on rebuilding her work life, my patient Terri had lost touch with an ecumenical contemplative group she'd participated in for twenty years. Out of the blue, Sandra, a colleague who had become a very close friend when they met at the beginning of their careers, called and suggested she join her in attending a candlelight vigil for peace during the upcoming holidays. Terri declined. It was across town in Atlanta, and was to start at 6:00 P.M.; traffic would be at a standstill. Terri's attempt to build her own graphic design firm outside of the corporate umbrella she was used to working within was taking longer than she'd hoped, and a low-grade, pervasive anxiety over future income meant she was working more hours than she should. The stress was chipping away at her sharpness and creativity; she was forgetting the lessons of self-care she had once known to restore her powers. She couldn't remember the last time she had taken a real vacation.

During the days after the call from Sandra, a persistent sensation dogged Terri that something had been missing in her life. It felt physical as memories of Sandra's and her search for meaning, something beyond what they'd valued in their early lives, began to activate her brain circuits of connection. At the last minute, Terri realized she desperately wanted to attend the vigil. She'd been working hard and mostly alone for so many years, and she was once again hungry for what the group had to offer. She decided to go. Looking up at the clock, she hesitated; there was no way she would make it on time. But a wave of determination—she didn't know where it came from—pushed her to override the urge to give up, sit back down, and turn her attention to work. She stood up, packed her things, and left the office.

The decisions Terri seemed to be making consciously were happening in concert with an activated brain and nervous system. By the time she reached for her car's door handle, she was receiving strong, contradictory signals simultaneously urging her onward and making navigation difficult: eager to get there, stressed over arriving late. It's the same push-pull we get when we are really hungry for breakfast but running late and need to get out the door quickly. Hijacked by the stress of haste, the brain is less able to focus on the small actions needed to make breakfast. Hence opening the box of oatmeal while rushing to grab the blueberries, both spilling, a lamp knocked over while stumbling to reach for the vacuum, errant feet smashing blueberries into the kitchen floor. The mishaps pile up, causing more stress and further delay.

In response to Terri's feeling both lonely and anxious about being late, her hypothalamus and pituitary fired up the adrenal glands to send out stress hormones to stimulate vigilance in the face of danger. The amygdala, the brain's fear center, came online too strongly, clouding her judgment and overpowering the vagus nerve's ability to keep heart rate and blood pressure in the sweet spot of well-being. Terri hated the idea of missing something and hated the idea of disturbing others, especially when she hadn't been around the group for the last four or five years.

In the right amount, stress hormones can make us alert and eager to learn; but combined with low blood sugar, financial worry, and a nervous system deprived of a sense of belonging, levels of cortisol and adrenaline were just high enough to make Terri feel jittery and confused. With the emotional amygdala cutting off pathways to the calmer frontal lobe—the seat of higher reason—she lost focus and swung a left a block too early. The GPS app showed her arrival would be delayed another ten minutes.

By the time Terri pulled into the poorly lit parking lot, her stress system was on fire, activating inflammation, the body's response to infections and wounds, as well as an overdose of cortisol and adrenaline, which is what the hypothalamus and adrenals throw at us when our sense of well-being and belonging are shaken. If inflammation goes unnoticed and unchecked, it lays the foundation for heart disease, cancer, diabetes, loss of memory, and decreased cognitive functioning.

When Terri finally opened the door to the meditation hall, the flames from the candles held by some of the participants were creating a soft glow. As she took in the low light, the spiritual icons, the Gregorian chant rising from hidden speakers around the comfortably full room, her body absorbed the signal of safety, which calmed the adrenals and brought the brain's vagus nerve—the body's largest—online to begin settling her heart rate, blood pressure, and hormones of threat. Inflammation would now have a chance to calm.

As hands reached out in greeting while she searched for an open spot, the brain's reward center activated. The hormones of bonding, such as oxytocin, and feel-good chemicals like the dopamine we get in surges from orgasm and deep conversation, streamed into her body as she felt enfolded by familiar and unfamiliar hugs. Oxytocin was modulating her brain's stress response, signaling the hypothalamus and pituitary to stand down in their call for energy from the adrenals. She was beginning the recovery process. Endorphins, the same neurochemicals that trigger a runner's high, were released as the peace and good-hearted intentions of those in the room cooled her system. Through connection, Terri's brain was beginning to connect the neural pathways to contentment.

Her nervous system was beginning to allow her to be present, to think clearly, to shift her attention from worry about her work and the logistics of the day to connecting with a community and its larger purpose. Her memory of so many years of feeling like she belonged in this room stimulated the hypothalamus to release oxytocin to be received by specialized receptors in the brain's nucleus accumbens, which in turn sent signals to other pathways to release a flood of serotonin, the neurochemical of wellbeing. The deep enjoyment of connection began to flood Terri's being once again. She was feeling more like herself with every passing moment, more like the "Me" she had been accustomed to experiencing.

The feeling that had dogged her earlier in the week, that something was missing, was a craving for the feeling of being present with a group, the feeling of her mirror neurons helping her to reflect the peace and well-being of others in a known community. Her body was seeking the stimulation of the neurochemicals of familiarity. That Terri would arrive home feeling calmer, more peaceful, more alert, more friendly, more hopeful and creative, is not a psychological or spiritual mystery. It's a brain and nervous system response to the cascade of neurohormones essential to the well-being of the social animal, *Homo sapiens*. It's a response to the familiar feeling of the tent of "Me."

Think for a minute about where the label of "Me" falls when you say it out loud. When we are young, a simple declaration of "I am" seems to do the trick. As we take on different responsibilities, our identity may feel powered by various roles—wife, employee, doctor, mother, friend, activist, caretaker—where we fit into our communities, with which friends and family members we feel we belong. Depending on circumstances, life may force us to question whether any of these things are "Me." Do I feel like "Me" without my kids at home, without a spouse? Do I feel like "Me" living outside the city and home in which I have lived for thirty years? Do I feel like "Me" without my job of more than three decades, without the co-workers and friends who have defined my social life? If not, then what happened to the "Me" that felt so certain? It may feel, in the second half, as though your tent is emptying. Trying to refill it may not always prompt the best choices.

Tricks and Traps of Refilling the Tent

Loneliness, defined by having fewer relationships in which you feel heard and understood than you need to maintain a basic sense of well-being, has become a big enough epidemic that more than sixty million Americans say it's a major source of unhappiness in their lives. The culprit, it turns out, may not be loneliness but the lack of a sense of belonging. This is what happens when the sense of "Me" contracts as a result of kids moving out, friends and loved ones moving away or passing away, leaving the home and community in which we raised a family, careers ending and roles changing; it's as though the tent of "Me" becomes empty of belonging. These chronic feelings of not belonging can drive a cascade of biological events that accelerate the aging process, even increasing the risk of dementia. It shows up in the stress hormones, immune function, and cardiovascular function, and some research is suggesting that it can cut your life span by as much as fifteen years.

Knowing this now, Sherry is working hard to shift internally. "I can't afford to move back east at this point, though if I could, I'd do it in a heartbeat. But I learned I have to fight the urge to curl up at home. Whenever I gave in, I started drinking too much," she confessed. Alcohol had not been a big problem in the past. "But it got to a point that it was threatening my relationship with David. And I can understand. He was protecting his family."

Sherry used the brain's wiring for social connection to turn things around and repopulate her tent of "Me." "I've started to take exercise classes," she told me, scrunching up her face, "which I used to hate, but they give me a chance to meet new people. I've made a few new walking buddies that way. And I'm volunteering to take meals to people who are housebound. Seeing the struggles of so many not much older than I am puts things in perspective. I have no choice but to stop feeling sorry for myself."

Connection in real time, even virtually, with longtime friends, family, and colleagues, reminds the nervous system that *Yes, I am still "me."* The brain's insula, in its scan to ascertain the body's well-being, will engage in helping to confirm that *I still feel the same patterns; my mirror neurons are stimulated to react in the same way; my systems are receiving feedback that I still matter.* When the insula gets a response it isn't used to, the alarm bells ring. It can drive compensatory behaviors through a cascade of neurohormones to create a craving for familiarity. It can take the form of an impulse to drink or overeat; or after the end of a long relationship, it can reawaken all those adolescent brain circuits for pursuing bad boys. It depends on what kind of familiarity the nervous system is craving.

Toxic Familiarity

At first, after her divorce at fifty-seven, Rena had a hard time finding someone to connect with. "I don't understand, Louann," she said to me, "because it's not for lack of availability. There is not a shortage of men to date, and many of them at this age want to get serious. They all want to remarry. But somehow, there's just no spark for me with any of them. And if there is, it keeps hitting a dead end."

Knowing Rena's history, this made sense. Her father had been an alcoholic. Dennis, her husband of twenty years, had gambled in secret, and if I had to diagnose him from afar, I'd say he was also a narcissist. For twenty-seven years, Rena did a dance responding to his incessant demands that she be responsible for making his world perfect. No matter what she said or did, it was wrong. She was constantly accused of being selfish, of not considering his feelings, of not wanting to make him happy. "It got to the point that when he asked me my opinion, I would ask him, 'What would you like me to say?' And of course that would send him into a rage," Rena said. "And I started to get scared for my safety. His temper was becoming extreme, and he would chase me around the house yelling. I used to go to the guest room and lock the door." Years later I could see how sad she still was about how things ended. "A part of me still feels like it's my fault."

Over the next two years, Rena found herself dating again. She fell for a couple of men just like Dennis. She felt instant chemistry with them, lots of excitement at the beginning. When friends set her up with really nice guys who weren't narcissists, she felt like there was no magic and didn't call them back.

Through her childhood and long marriage, Rena's nervous system had been trained to crave an unreasonable and demanding partner. The familiarity made her feel alive. Lack of familiar triggering will make a safe setting feel boring or uninteresting. When we are used to being continually activated by a rage-aholic, the state of fear becomes equivalent to feeling alive and like "me." When we don't feel that, we feel bored and adrift. The nervous system signals the brain to search for meaning by connecting with familiarity; this is one of the reasons that even after a spouse has stopped drinking and is sober, things don't *feel* right. Rena had her work cut out for her, and it would take some time to help her rebalance.

Toxic familiarity is poison to the brain's sense of self, deepening familiar patterns that send self-destructive signals to the brain. In the reproductive phase, we can muscle through a lot of misery. But in the second half, the stress of things going badly is more apparent, and the opportunity to wake up to the symptoms is more available than at any other time in our lives. The social stress circuits become more sensitive as women get older because the HPA (hypothalamic, pituitary, adrenal) axis responds more quickly to social stress but takes more time and attention to calm and reset. While we recognize more readily through experience that we can't demand perfection from ourselves or our friends—that would leave us quite alone and isolated—we can also recognize that if the stress of a specific relationship is paralyzing, it's time to reconsider the connection. Terri was finally, miraculously, ready to do just that. In the Upgrade our lives no longer have to include familiar experiences that lock us into toxic patterns.

Resetting the Nervous System

One patient of mine, Jean, who lost her husband to cancer when she was seventy-four, didn't call anyone for months. Somehow, in her mind-numbing isolation, she became convinced that because her husband died of cancer, she was an unlovable failure whom no one would want to see. The thought was entirely irrational and had nothing to do with reality. But the incorporation of her husband into the tent of "Me" meant that when that piece of her was gone, she interpreted its absence as inadequacy. "It's like every voice that ever told me I wasn't good enough, that made me feel incompetent, came roaring back to fill the space that Jack left. I know now, after talking it through, that it was crazy, but that's how it felt," she told me.

Through nervous system harmonization, we physically incorporate the people we are close to. You don't realize it's like singing in harmony until your choirmate is gone. What we feel in their absence is the nervous system and brain patterns being stuck on a search for the familiar.

Luckily friends were persistent in their efforts to help Jean get back into the world. It took years for her nervous system to recalibrate in the healing space of belonging. "I'll never get over it," she said, and I encouraged her to allow that visceral sense of loss. It's impossible to replace the people we lose. "But I can see a way forward," she concluded.

Acts of social withdrawal are a razor's edge. When we need to calm agitation, rest, and refresh the nervous system, a little alone time can be good. But there is a tipping point of solitude that increases agitation. Belonging is one of the best ways to calm the nervous system in the long run.

Even a pleasant exchange with a stranger provides the nervous system with the essential affirmation that we matter. These exchanges can help balance us cognitively.

This is why solitary confinement is so cruel. We mirror others, so when we are off, a balanced nervous system can reset us, just by being in proximity. We can reset one another or we can destabilize one another. We all know that friend we should not call when we are fragile, or that person we should call when we are fragile, or that fragile friend we know we can help reset. It's not mystical or weird; it's the neuroscience of mirror neurons and oxytocin, which attune us to one another through body language, vocal inflection, and a million tiny, unconscious cues.

Think about what it feels like when you are out to dinner or at someone's home with a bunch of friends. Remember the rapid-fire conversations, the group laughter, the food, the one-on-one connections. If you close your eyes and allow yourself to pull up a strong memory, chances are it's making you happy. That feeling is good for your nervous system and good for your brain. If you visualize yourself at a party from your youth, turning on the music you heard then and dancing as if the room were filled with your oldest and best friends, there is evidence that it has a positive impact on memory, physical strength, vision, and hearing.

When we lack social stimulation, whether it's actual or imagined, parts of us wither. Without its counterbalance, we lose those essential brain vitamins of social connection and with them our resolve and resilience. In isolation after her retirement as an executive assistant, Pauline started reexperiencing hurt she thought she had set aside decades earlier. Old pain from her marriage, even her childhood, began to resurface. It wasn't just because of the lack of distraction through a schedule that was no longer full; it was the lack of nourishment via oxytocin and serotonin for the brain circuits that help us remain in the zone of well-being. In the second half of life, that zone narrows, its borders become more porous, and the signals that we are out of it are stronger; we can become suddenly overwhelmed in ways that feel paralyzing. It was helping her granddaughter move to Los Angeles that made her feel connected and useful again.

The experience of reciprocity that happens when we are a part of a circle of others feels good to the brain and nervous system. Mirror neurons and oxytocin play a huge role in how we regulate one another. In a harmonious group, mirror neurons ping signals of happiness and belonging among the members. The bond is reinforced and rewarded by oxytocin sent from the hypothalamus to the nucleus accumbens bringing one of the brain's calming and pain relieving systems online with a cocktail of serotonin, dopamine, and other endorphins that are like a balm of instant well-being to the brain and body's nerves.

The presence of trust and a calmer nervous system means heightened cognitive powers are retained longer. It also means a longer life, as the immune system is allowed to function properly instead of reacting to signals of threat stimulated by an isolation-activated stress system. Trust and hugs become like rainy-day funds to use in moments of stress. They create our reserve for meeting life's ups and downs with flexibility and strength, the resilience that helps us return to our optimal emotional and physical zone of well-being in the Upgrade.

The correlation between social connection and long-term benefits for brain, heart, and systemic health is strong. By lowering stress hormones, social connection reduces inflammation, improving cognition and immune function. Through stimulation of feel-good neurochemicals, we become motivated to engage in healthier habits. The feeling of care coming from others helps us engage in self-care.

Belonging is like jet fuel for any habit that supports good health and well-being; it's as essential to improving cognition and decreasing risk of diabetes as getting enough sleep. New research is showing that isolation is likely to be as damaging to health as smoking, lack of exercise, or a poor diet. While it shortens a woman's life span by as much as fifteen years, those who feel supported by their spouses to go out in groups of three or more girlfriends twice a week live years longer.

Trust, one of the key ingredients of belonging, feels good to the brain and nervous system. Because of changing hormones in the Transition and Upgrade, we again have a unique opportunity to break free of misplaced trust. Before the Transition, a hug even from a partner you distrusted would trigger a release of oxytocin, making you forget every suspicion.

I used to warn a woman before the Transition not to let her partner hug her if she suspected him or her of lying. A hug would set off a flood of oxytocin, boosted by spiking levels of estrogen, that would make her believe whatever she was told.

In the Upgrade, we get the best of both worlds. We can still lead with love and trust, but with constant lower estrogen, our thinking is no longer overwhelmed by big surges of oxytocin. Trust becomes a choice, rather than a neurohormonal destiny. We have the ability to notice when the nervous system is tugged by a familiar yet unhealthy nervous-system pattern of another.

Giving the brain the essential vitamins of connection and validation is key to the Upgrade. For just a moment I'm going to ask you to put aside your pride in independence and your denial of aging. Ladies, if you are leaking, if you're accusing everyone of mumbling, or if you've got back pain, chances are you are going to start saying no to invitations. Stop it. Just stop it. If you can't walk well, get the damn scooter you've been resisting. Sixty percent of women over sixty have a mobility problem, so I know I am talking to some of you. If you think everyone around you is suddenly speaking too softly, go to the doctor and get your hearing tested. Stubbornness born of pride is one of the biggest obstacles to optimizing the Upgrade. Do everything you can to stay connected.

It's not just longevity we are after in the Upgrade; it's joy, emotional strength, and sharpness. Who we are arises in a context, not in isolation. Who we are is a composite formed out of connection; our interaction with others is the ground on which we plant the tent pole that supports our sense of self. Engaging in healthy connection isn't an optional part of life, something that we do when we have extra time; it's intrinsic to who we are as humans. Finding belonging is not a frivolous, secondary activity. It determines whether we enter a downgrade or an Upgrade.

As we move into the Upgrade, whom we surround ourselves with becomes more important in the tent of "Me 2.0." Find those who help you discover the best in yourself. Immerse yourself among those who are on the same quest in the renovation of their tent of "Me." As part of its evolution, the human brain became primed for living in groups, and the bonding hormone, oxytocin, cemented the need. All these millennia later, the evidence for this primal need is confirmed by studies that show girl-friends improve our health. So head out or video-chat with a group of four; for full health and stress-reduction benefits, drop any trace of guilt. And to amplify those benefits, set aside all your responsibilities and take a trip with the ladies. In times of stress, the female brain, even after the Upgrade, releases oxytocin for bonding, not just the stress hormone cor-tisol, which makes us flee or fight. In the Upgrade we seek out bonds with others who give us permission to be totally ourselves.

Upgrading the Mommy Brain

Chapter 8

"Seriously, she got a headline alert that there was a blizzard coming, and my mom found it necessary to stop what she was doing at work in Dallas, pick up the phone, and call me in Chicago to remind me to wear my gloves and hat," says thirty-five-year-old communications executive La-tanya. "Does she really think I'm still ten?"

We may have helped push them out of the house to live independent lives, but whether or not we ever push them out of our tent of "Me" is a separate question. But it may be a necessary step if you want to keep them in your lives. As my son will attest, too many of these kinds of inter-ferences will mean our adult children begin to shut us out. And those moments or days when they don't return our texts or calls can feel like part of us is left hanging in the breeze, slowly being ripped away by the wind. I have found it utterly defeating how tied to the moods of my son I still am.

When the mommy-brain circuits turn on, it changes who you are. The passage of the baby's head through the cervix and vagina triggers a surge of oxytocin, as does nipple stimulation during nursing; but skin-to-skin contact and the smell of the top of the baby's head alone initiate a powerful cascade of bonding hormones. Through motherhood we are re-wired to detect the smell of their bodies and the smell of their poop, hear the different sounds of their cries as their very being gets incorporated into our tent of "Me." Whether you gave birth to the child or not doesn't matter: Skin-to-skin contact changes everything.

No matter how quickly they've grown up, no matter how old we are, the mommy-brain circuits are very hard to turn off. My brain is hijacked by those mommy circuits frequently, even though my son is now an adult. When Whitney first moved out of the house, I used to go into his room to smell his smell. Lately I have to practice hard to cultivate loving detach-ment, because at a certain point, our kids really wish our mommy brains would leave them alone to live their lives.

Even if our kids are doing well, we will still worry. Our frontal lobes are always on for problem solving. Though everything may be okay, our overthinking and overconcern will create problems where they don't exist, pushing us to interfere and rescue when there is no crisis to be rescued from. For that, our kids have the most powerful weapons: distance, si-lence, and separation. Regardless of age, the female brain's circuitry is still wired for connection. Their silence is DEFCON 1 to the female brain and its nervous system. Jane Isay writes honestly and deftly of her experience in her book *Walking on Eggshells*:

> There were some rocky years when I thought I'd lost him and he didn't want to hear anything I had to say. Very painful. He had to teach me how to separate from him. I had to learn to pay more attention to myself and less to him. I had to become accustomed to living on the periphery of his life. I had no power and had to learn (still learning) to give up expectations. It turns out he is a lot of fun and is witty, knowledgeable and smart. It has taken me years to adjust to the new normal. And challenges still come up all the time. We keep on trying to stay close to each other without driving each other crazy. Accepting my own mistakes and failings— which he and I laugh at together now. I know he loves me and occasionally he will even tell me.

When Whitney pushed back against how often I was stopping by his apartment, I said, "I want to see you a lot because I think you're lonely." He responded, "Yes, I am lonely, but seeing you isn't going to do anything about it." I thought my presence was giving him someone to hang out with. If anything, the opposite was true. My anxious presence was keeping him from exploring how to address his own loneliness. Showing me that let me off the hook. I was no longer responsible for addressing his wounds.

For the relationship with our adult children to survive, we have to expand the mommy circuits to a broader target. If we keep hovering, their experience is that we don't respect them or validate their adulthood. And if we don't find a way to validate their adulthood, they will erect a wall. They will block us on social media, screen our calls, or simply be dishonest with us. They will find their own ways to push our relationship with them to a place they can tolerate, even if it hurts us. Trust me.

For the majority of women who have become mothers, the mommy brain has dominated our adult reality, motivated by the urgent need to keep them alive until they are eighteen. Our social lives and work lives revolved around getting them to the right place at the right time, connecting with the school and other moms, engaging in a daily game of high-level calendar chess. But that's about as far ahead as we've thought. In the sweep of history, female survival beyond the fertility phase is new. The completely absorbing balancing act of job, social life, and children's activities that hijacks the brain and nervous system is over. There is no road map to transitioning into being a mother of adult children. In the new era of longevity, this territory has to be mapped, this developmental phase has yet to be named or explored.

You've probably heard the story of the old man walking through the woods who comes across a butterfly struggling to get out of its cocoon. He thinks the butterfly is stuck, and so he opens the cocoon. The butterfly has shriveled wings and a fat body and is unable to fly, leaving it more vulnerable to birds looking for a meal. The struggle to break the cocoon is what makes the wings strong and the body smaller. The old man's instinct to rescue deprived the butterfly of its birthright: strength to fly.

I don't know where the story comes from, but I've heard it told many times by various people. Learning when not to open the cocoon for our kids is as important to them now as when we would reassure them they were okay after a fall on the playground. We can give our adult children their own dignity by treating them as we would other adults.

One sign of a mommy brain in a downgrade is thinking we know our kids. We don't. We can honor them by giving them space, and that is how we will get to know them as adults. In the Upgrade, we approach them as if we were getting to know a new friend, listening rather than interrogating: Did you pay the bill? Where is the form you were supposed to fill out? Did you call the dentist? Leave them alone. They will figure it out, or grow from the consequences if they don't.

The transition into the second half of life is a long shift into letting go, practicing loving detachment, remaining silent to listen to adult kids, spouses, and siblings. We learn the hard way that things grow best when they are tended lightly and learn to hold the space for our loved ones as opposed to marking and guarding the perimeter of their sandbox. It's not easy to stop being at the ready to lay down our lives for them. It's not easy to keep from violating the space we formerly felt entitled to enter through interrogation. We would never cross that line with other adults we know; the questions would be disrespectful. And rescue-mommy-brain mode only makes them feel disempowered.

Extreme Mommy-Brain Challenges

It takes love and humility to accept our own weaknesses and to come to terms with the failings of our children.

—*Jane Isay,* Walking on Eggshells

If you are the mother of an adult child with a self-destructive habit like alcohol or drugs, or one with a mental health issue for which they have opted not to follow treatment, how you deal with the incorporation of your child into your tent of "Me" can have a dramatic impact on your own life.

"I was at the end of my financial rope," Wendy, sixty-four, told me after a talk I gave in Denver. "I come from rural Nebraska and I grew up very poor. But I was lucky enough to go to college and be very successful in the financial industry. My husband and I made a lot of money together, and so when Chris, our oldest of three kids, became ill with his addiction at fifteen, we started writing six-figure checks to rehab facilities. He was in five different in-house programs by the time he was twenty-two." I could see and feel her pain. As a psychiatrist, I know that the recovery rate for addicts and alcoholics is barely 30 percent. The vast majority never get out from under their disease. And as a doctor familiar with these programs, I also know that Wendy was telegraphing that they had spent more than a million dollars on various facilities.

"After my husband died five years ago," Wendy continued, "I just didn't know what to do. I had retired and needed to make sure the money we'd saved was going to last. I also have another son and daughter and wanted to be able to help them when they needed it. But Chris kept getting into trouble, and as a mother, what do you say to your child when he's in pain and he's begging you for help?"

When we have incorporated another into our tent of "Me," whether a spouse or child or close friend, the nervous system sends us powerful alerts when something is wrong in their lives or they are trying to create distance. It's this unconscious intertwining of our nervous system with theirs that can keep us hooked to people who can cause us damage. We become codependent, literally addicted to them. The nervous system seeks familiarity and repetition. It seems weird, but if we are used to someone making us miserable, we will oddly crave the familiar misery unless we find the strength, the friends, and the support to help us break the cycle. We will need help. (See appendix, page 274.) Because while it feels bad to keep toxic loved ones in our tent of "Me," it can feel worse to push them out. The dilemma can send us into isolation as we push away those who challenge our addiction to their problems. We don't have a road map for dealing with this. If we have even a tiny ounce of the instinct for self-preservation, it will kick our social circuits back into gear; almost against our own desire, it will push us out of the house to at least browse in a department store, talk to a salesperson, call a therapist, take up an invitation to a dinner with a group of people we might not normally seek out. If we can't hear or don't honor those impulses, the nervous system will pull us down the rabbit hole of obsession into intractable melancholy.

"By the time I looked up from my relationship with Chris," Wendy said, "I was completely alone. Other parents would talk about how great their kids were doing. I didn't know how to relate to people without talking about his problems, and I didn't know how to be present with others without checking for his texts or making sure he was still alive. I would feel jealous their kids were doing great. It made me testy and unpleasant to be around. My nervous system was so wired to his well-being that I no longer had a life or even a sense of myself. I was on my knees."

Different people are drawn to different tools for addressing isolation and repairing the tent of "Me." "I started with Al-Anon," Wendy told me about her decision to make a change. "I worked the program as hard as I could to learn how to make that separation with my son and start to care for myself. Two years ago I did the hardest thing I've ever done in my life. I changed my phone number and moved. I didn't tell Chris how to find me. I had to finally come to grips with the reality that I am powerless to help him. I've let him go at thirty-five. Keeping him close was keeping me from living, it was damaging my relationship with my other two kids, and it was keeping him from finding help. I had to get out of his way and let him walk his own path. My other kids were worried about what Chris's illness was doing to me, especially the times he physically threatened me. By the time I made the decision, I had lost touch with most of my friends. Anyone outside of Al-Anon had no way of understanding the hell I was living."

The nervous system is trained to respond and behave habitually by our social connections. So if our nervous system has been engaged with the toxic familiarity of a loved one who is addicted, mentally ill, or is a rage-aholic, breaking those connections within the tent of "Me" can feel apocalyptic. In the first weeks and months after that kind of separation, anxious boredom often sets in. "I didn't know what to do with myself after I moved and got settled in," Wendy told me. "I was so used to organizing my entire being around Chris's needs that disconnecting felt like an identity crisis. I didn't know who I was without the chaos." Wendy's nervous system was craving familiarity, and it was hard for her not to fill that void by becoming a codependent crisis machine, looking for or creating drama where there wasn't any.

When the tent of "Me" is unconsciously ensnared by the profound disorder of a child, it short-circuits the Upgrade. But as we grow more conscious of how the nervous system and brain can become a source of feedback in forming the tent of "Me," we can take more control over whom we let in and how much influence they get. Wendy realized that not only had she given Chris a place of prominence within her tent, but "I let him take over the tent pole. It was like he had control over how I judged myself and how I set my daily priorities. I was always reacting to something, a phone call or visit from him or a crisis, so I couldn't plan and was always canceling things. Yet at the time, it felt like it was the right way to be. Now I know I need to focus on self-care."

The Upgrade is our chance to radiate strength and goodness powered by the wisdom and courage to hold the space for whatever is emerging for the adult child. It takes patience. It will hurt when they lash out from pain. But once they hold their proper place in our tent of "Me," their unhappiness with us is no longer an identity-threatening pain. We can finally hold the space for ourselves and for them, in healthy, intimate separation.

Granny Brain

"The biggest hit of euphoria and the biggest speed bump in my family relationships showed up as the grandkids appeared on the scene," Ceci told me over our regular coffee.

I had wanted to know what had most challenged her stability in the Upgrade. "That's interesting," I said, feeling a little puzzled. I don't have grandchildren yet, so I have to rely on what I know from neuroscience and the experiences of others. "You hear all the time about the joy. A friend from Brazil always jokes that children are a necessary evil for getting grandchildren. But tell me about the challenges."

"When I held those babies," Ceci continued, "I thought my heart would burst. I never knew how big that love could be. It broke me open. The pull to be around my grandkids is so strong; our conversations as they grow up are so intimate, so filled with unconditional acceptance, so much mutual respect, so much deep listening. I'm in love. It's the only way to describe it."

The echoes of mommy-brain circuits are powerful, and even with lower levels of bonding hormones, they are easily reactivated. The blessing of the biological distance makes room for a more unconditional love, free of the fears, responsibility, and judgments we had with our own kids. The brain's nervous system doesn't incorporate them into the tent of "Me" with the same sense of daily urgency as it does our own children, so it's easier to approach their suffering with an open heart, ready to listen instead of going into control mode, fixing, and interfering. Still, the bond is shatteringly powerful.

This is the reactivation of the caretaking circuits pounded into the female brain and nervous system from the first years of life, the flood of oxytocin, the comfy, cozy progesterone, the nervous system's memory of the pleasurable part of bonding. There can be peace in those echoes, and clearly Ceci was experiencing that. "This sounds so great, Ceci. It's hard to imagine the downside."

"It's there," she replied. "You learn about it pretty suddenly: the first time you say no to your kids when they ask you to take a grandchild for a day or overnight. I said yes a lot after my first one was born. But then I started to feel like I was losing access to the goals I had set out for this period of my life. I'm still working pretty hard, and it's exhausting taking care of active grandkids. I want time for walks, for thinking, for rest, for reevaluating life, priorities, choices. If I am growing consciously into a better person, I can be better for everyone. If I can find peace and happiness, that will make a difference to others around me. It took a long time to understand, to really deeply get that my happiness is not selfish—it's a contribution to the happiness of others. I don't mean that small thing of being satisfied. I mean the big happiness that comes when you drop your worries about looks, clothes, money, possessions. When you can embrace life's joys and its scary uncertainties. That's the kind of centering and strengthening of my tent pole I am engaging in. This is my time for that. I'm worth it. And I have the right to claim it."

I could sense her now-or-never urgency, a feeling of breaking out of prison. And that might be just the right analogy.

By the time most girls are a year old, we are handed our first dolly and told to feed it with a fake bottle. The culture is already grooming us to become martyr moms, irrevocably and primarily responsible for the survival of our families. We are being prepared for what can at times feel like a prison of expectation and obligation, one we happily accept out of love but also in order to avoid the social price and guilt we pay for not complying. But in the second half, in the Upgrade, we can break that chain: We are no longer primarily responsible for the survival of small children, though society and the echoes of old wiring will try to tell us otherwise.

Martyr-mom wiring is very hard to undo. The shift to being centered comes when we are able to be alert to and resist the tug of the imprints of old waves, when we can shift our goals for the tent of "Me" from outward approval to our own well-being, making sure that we are meeting our best interests in a way that actually makes us better to and for everyone around us.

"So when I claim that time," Ceci said, "or I am busy with work and I say no, you'd think by my son or daughter's reaction that I had just said I hate them all and never want to see them again. You can't imagine the nasty things they say. 'Why am I not surprised. You were never there for us as kids. Why would I think you'd be any different as a grandmother?' They don't say these things to their father when he says no. And they don't ask him as often as they ask me."

"Wow, that's rough," I said. "There are a lot of emotions that are bound to come up, but how does that feel, viscerally, that tug of grandchildren and the anger of your kids?"

"For a long time it was like the first gun going off in the biggest internal battle I've ever fought." Ceci paused, sadness coming over her face. "Those caretaking impulses are real. The guilt over not acting on them is powerful." Seeing as women end up with 78 percent of all caretaking duties, data backs up her feeling. "And the things my kids say cut deep. But I go back to that tent metaphor you use. I have really been looking at who is controlling my tent pole. It got clear to me during my morning walks, which I started taking alone a couple times a week instead of with my group. As I upped my activity and felt stronger, I started to see that I wasn't the one always in control of my tent pole. I started to see who I had given access to. And it was a big shock. My kids, my friends, even my dead mother was still tugging on it. So I walked, exercised, did yoga, some writing and breathing exercises. All of that helped me see what was going on."

Because I'm in Charge!

I've known Diane through the medical community for years. She's an internist who is winding down her practice. She's been married for thirty-seven years—she met her partner in med school—has two kids in their twenties, and like many, cares for nearby aging parents. She's always been busy taking care of everybody's needs, and it hasn't always been easy getting a spot on her schedule. But she's been more available lately and I wondered what had changed. "It's easy to feel pulled in a million directions," she said. "It's easy to fall into the caretaking trap and just not have a life. . . ." Her voice trailed off as she looked at a message on her Apple Watch. "Hang on. Josh just texted me to say he lost his passport."

I knew her twenty-six-year-old son was traveling in Europe, and I was already moving toward my car keys to get out of her way. She had always been intensely involved in her kids' lives and I assumed our visit was over. "Oh no!" I said. "Do you have to go call him?"

"Absolutely not," she said, to my surprise. "I'll be right back." Diane disappeared into the kitchen and emerged with her phone. She appeared unmoved. "So what happened?" I asked.

As she handed me a cup of tea, she said, "I texted back and said, 'You're an adult. I'm sure you can find people at the airport to help you figure it out.'"

I was impressed. I am not confident I would be able to show the same restraint; my son pulls hard at my tent pole, and if I don't respond to what I perceive as his crises, then something doesn't feel quite right.

"Two years ago," she said, seeing the question arising in my face, "I would have said goodbye to you and run to his rescue. But that kind of behavior was crippling him and exhausting me. Same for my mom, who calls me obsessively. I answered every call no matter what I was in the middle of. So I found some things to keep her occupied and I stopped picking up the phone when she calls, which is literally every hour and a half. When I didn't answer, she started texting more, and I could see what was urgent and what wasn't. Not answering felt at first like a betrayal, and then I understood I was actually breaking an addiction. Kinda like code-pendency. As for my husband, I have learned to ignore any question emanating from the kitchen that begins with 'Where's the . . .' or 'How do I . . .' Somehow, he manages to find whatever he's looking for all by himself. I just have to sit on my hands until it passes."

Before the Transition you may have felt that it was just fine to let a whole bunch of people control your tent pole and that many things were your responsibility to fix: people, situations, the lives and relationships of others. That fixing impulse was a big part of the tent of "Me." It gave us confidence in our competence and our agency, until the day our plan didn't work, or it backfired. In the face of something going wrong comes a deflation of our sense of power and control, bringing on anxiety, fear, agitation, sadness; a collapse, whole or partial, of the tent of "Me." By pursuing what we can't fix, we get constant failure feedback in the tent of "Me."

In the Upgrade, we recognize that our tent pole doesn't belong to anyone else, and we can see there is little we can do to fix the minds of others. There is only one mind and one tent pole for which we must care: our own. After decades of trying to control others, acceptance of the truth of powerlessness over most everything frees us to finally know ourselves. I'm hoping that by the time I go, my son will agree that my epitaph will be "Finally learned to mind her own business." I'm still working on that.

The Relationship Brain

Chapter 9

*The biggest predictor of how healthy you will be at eighty
is your satisfaction with your relationships at fifty.*

From birth, the female brain is a mean, lean, observing machine. The ability to read faces and hear vocal inflection can make women seem like mind readers, all because of an awesomely fine-tuned nervous system and the right mix of neurochemicals to support this particular talent. By now, you've probably spent a lifetime perfecting your ability to anticipate the needs and moods of others. You can feel their exhaustion, hunger, or sadness before they do, and before you know it, you've set about trying to fix the problem. Part of that ability is societal—experiments have shown that anyone in a subordinate position develops this skill—and part of it is hardwired into us as women.

It can be powerful, having this ability, and it can be exhausting.

I was thinking about Sylvia and Robert, the couple we followed in *The Female Brain*. Their long marriage had broken up, but I was curious to know if while married she had felt what so many of the women I knew also experienced during long partnerships. It's the feeling of absorbing your partner's nervous system to the point that it seems to drown out your own nervous system's signals—a kind of extreme empathy. "I always had a hard time not physically feeling my husband's emotions," Sylvia, now seventy-seven, told me. "I would walk into a room, and if he were down and feeling angry, I got a knot in my stomach. I could feel the gripping in my chest and sweat in my palms when he was anxious or angry. I could also feel his contentment and peace, so that was a plus. But for the most part I kept feeling like I'd lost my center, that I couldn't feel my own emotions, my own discomfort. I had a split in my soul. It felt like I didn't have a self that wasn't absorbed in his reality."

"That must have been really disconcerting," I said, having known the same feeling. Emotional contagion is a large field of study, and from the nervous-system side, our oxytocin and mirror neurons act as amplifiers for "catching" someone else's feelings. When you add the closeness of an intimate relationship, it's much harder to resist resonating with the emotional state of a loved one. "It was enraging, actually. After forty years I looked up and realized I knew him inside and out; but I had become a stranger to myself. It's part of why I left. I needed to find and stand on my own ground again."

In the beginning of an intimate relationship, the brain's love-attachment system, driven by neurohormones—more oxytocin in females, more vasopressin in males—is primed for us to take the habits, tastes, and preferences of the person to whom we are becoming attached as our own. As the tent of "Me" expands to include this new person and their feelings—their likes and dislikes, their experiences—how we feel in our skin is altered. When we or a spouse are away for a long business trip, that feeling of being out of sorts is a signal from the nervous system that some kind of essential feedback is missing. That first hug upon return so often sets things right, as it activates the calming circuits of belonging.

There is a flip side to this deep connectedness. Many times I've found myself holding attitudes or behaving in ways that don't feel native to me, attitudes and behaviors I might not be proud of. Neuroscience shows how many of our attitudes and habits and how much of our physiology come from what we absorb from those closest to us; what we think and say and do may not always be the real us, though it may feel like it in the moment.

This deep, unconscious absorption of another's nervous-system patterns is amplified during the fertility phase by estrogen: It makes orgasm more readily available and pumps much more oxytocin into our systems. The calming of those bonding and caretaking circuits during the Upgrade can give us more bandwidth for looking inward, for analyzing and focusing on what's necessary to do for ourselves. It can give us the strength to resist being pushed by the echoes of old caretaking waves that would have driven us to race to the rescue of everyone else. Especially when we begin to understand the neuroscience of empathy.

Empathy, feeling the feelings of another, is a gift at the heart of compassion. But according to studies at the Max Planck Institute in Germany and the University of Wisconsin at Madison, it has a potential dark side. That we feel what someone else feels, especially their suffering, sounds noble and virtuous. But think about what happens to us when we are faced with the suffering of those close to us, how easy it is to feel debilitating sadness over what they are going through, how easy it is to drown in their pain. We don't need to see the results of fMRI (functional MRI) studies to tell us that feeling someone else's suffering lights up the pain circuits in our own brains. This kind of passive resonance can easily slide into empathetic distress, a powerful nervous-system force that can release a tsunami of stress neurochemicals and overwhelm our ability to think clearly, function normally, or engage in helpful problem solving. Sylvia struggled with feeling porous to Robert's moods. So did Ceci with her ex-husband, and pretty much every woman I've ever spoken to who has been in a long-term partnership. I know that feeling myself with both my husband and son. Even in a healthy relationship, if we are swamped by a partner's depression, we won't be any good to ourselves or to them. The stress of another can wake up our fear-triggering amygdala; when that little almond-sized brain organ takes over, it cuts off access to clear thinking. We fly, hair on fire, into rescue-survival mode.

Finding nervous-system independence was becoming a crucial self-care issue for Sylvia. When we last left off with their story, Sylvia had found freedom in the Upgrade; she had started setting new boundaries and was determined to start a career in her midfifties. The changes in Sylvia frightened Robert, and their forty-year marriage began to unravel. She moved out and they divorced. I caught up with them again to see if anything had changed.

It turns out that after about six months, things cooled off enough that they could begin to rediscover their friendship. They dated other people, but when they had trouble, they still turned to each other. When Robert got a bad flu, Sylvia came over every day for two weeks to help him. When Sylvia's mother needed legal work, Robert continued to care for his former mother-in-law. His attempts at new relationships were unsuccessful. "I had a woman leave in the middle of dinner," Robert told me, "because she realized I was still in love with Sylvia. It was clear I was never going to be able to commit to anyone else. So I made a commitment to Sylvia to go back to therapy and see if we could work things out."

After seven years apart, Sylvia moved back in, and they joked with me about living in sin. They traveled the world and really enjoyed themselves. Sylvia continued her career, starting and running a mental health nonprofit and later handing it off to the next generation but still conducting workshops for families and educators. Robert kept practicing law but reduced the firm's capacity and moved his practice into the den.

Robert is fourteen years older than Sylvia, and his cognitive decline had a profound impact on her life. Sylvia was still traveling for work, but Robert steadily became more easily frightened and needier. He became obsessed with worry that Sylvia would leave again, especially for a younger man, so she traveled only with him. But as he became more frail, they stayed home.

Over time, as his memory worsened, he became more like the old Robert, griping and complaining all the time, not well enough to be fully independent but stubborn enough to insist he could take care of himself. His routine made him happy: breakfast in the kitchen, a couple of hours at the computer in his home office, lunch in the kitchen, news in the library the rest of the day. He could no longer hear the TV, so he read the ticker at the bottom. At four thirty he had a martini, fueling evening irritability and insomnia.

Sylvia tried everything to keep him engaged with the world, to see friends and family. As his memory slipped, she became more isolated, not only because she was trapped at home but because having a normal conversation was no longer an option. "I was losing my friend," she told me. "I couldn't talk to him about daily events or discuss politics. He couldn't retain memory for anything except the law. On that front, he was still sharp as a tack."

Sylvia was becoming depressed and angry, and though she herself is a mental health expert, and has recommended therapy for other women in similar situations, she believed she was handling things just fine. She couldn't see that she needed someone to talk to, someone with expertise in elders who are in the process of dementing, who could help her with strategies for retaining some of her own hard-won independence. That's when her daughter reached out to me again. Age was taking down Robert's cognition. The isolation and loneliness were threatening Sylvia's nervous system as well, turning her Upgrade into a downgrade.

I knew that in order to disconnect the nervous system from contagion with a partner's requires mind/body techniques for closing off circuitry and containing the tent of "Me." I asked Sylvia how she managed to separate, to remain connected to Robert but not be overwhelmed by his moods. "I was working with a yoga teacher who helped me recognize when my husband's emotions were too prominent in my tent of 'Me,'" Sylvia told me. When she felt pulled by Robert's emotions, Sylvia was taught to first consciously slow her breath and bring her attention to her belly, a point just below and behind the navel. Once she was able to feel that connection, she rested her mind lightly on that spot. By bringing her attention to the center of balance in her body, it helped her focus on remaining centered. And while her attention was occupied, it meant she was able to disconnect from the habit of searching for signals of distress coming from Robert; it meant she had the option not to be so reactive to them.

When Sylvia did her breathing and body-awareness meditation, her tent flap could gently close—not lock, just create enough of a seal to contain the nervous system's circuit relaying the visceral sense of self. "This is what I found keeps the integrity of me," Sylvia told me as she described how much more powerful she felt in this practice and how it made her better able to respond not only to her husband but also to the ups and downs of life circumstances.

I like to think of this process as remaining in my own Hula-Hoop. I use this image when I feel too pulled by my husband's emotions. So many of us have spent a lot of our energy trying to step inside other people's Hula-Hoops, fixing and managing what we find there. But doing that also takes away the dignity of their feelings and their autonomy. So staying within my circle—like the ones they painted on the ground in parks during the COVID-19 pandemic to set boundaries for physical distancing—means I'm supporting the integrity of myself and everyone else around me.

Change and the Fear Circuits

Sylvia's practice to disconnect from Robert's mood felt wrong to her at first. Any change, good or bad, can throw a system's homeostasis off. In the early stages of shifting to the Upgrade, the nervous system needs to get used to the new shape of the tent of "Me" and the new, firmer placement of the tent pole. Like learning any new skill, or inhabiting any new state, it takes practice. The new habits almost always feel wrong at first.

The brain on default evaluates change through a lens of fear. We are wired to scan for threat to normalcy, for an indication of the slightest thing being a little off, to be constantly alert to change, ready to interpret it as a possible threat to our lives. The process by which bad news burns so deeply into us is called negativity bias. It can be a good thing, triggering healthy fear to avoid real danger, and life-threatening if we ignore the fear signals. If we didn't have negativity bias, we would be like those who don't have pain receptors and burn themselves on a hot skillet. Yet it's important to remember every day that the brain is like Velcro for negativity and Teflon for positivity. When the brain detects change, the lack of familiarity breaks through as a 9-1-1 call. It's that same bias that can mistake a healthy change, as in perhaps dating someone who is different but better for us, for danger.

Before the Transition, with full-bloom hormone levels that drive us to seize the world, our discovery circuits, the dopamine and adrenaline rush of the new, overwhelm the fear of negativity bias. We muscle through, fueled by the high of the new and the next. But the Transition and Upgrade are different. The discovery circuits are quieter without the strong pulse of androgens like DHEA and testosterone. Perception of change can manifest as deep anxiety during the Transition. What feels dangerous now might not have felt dangerous in our late thirties and early forties.

Caution and hypervigilance are core parts of the wiring that develops in women through acculturation, but they aren't our natural state; they're the wiring that emerges in anyone in a subordinate position. We become hyperalert to the needs of the "boss," able to anticipate and ameliorate quickly to avoid what our cavewoman wiring perceives as a threat to our source of food, clothing, and shelter. We hold being always ready, willing, and able as the peak of a highly functioning, thriving female, but it's a time-limited coping skill whose wiring comes undone in the Transition. The opportunity is freedom from the feeling of being on call 24-7 to respond to the needs of others. Explaining this to Sylvia made her ready for this kind of freedom.

The Brain Benefits of Groups

The pressure we put on a one-on-one long partnership to serve so many of our needs may actually be damaging to cognition in the Upgrade. In a study on aging female mice at Ohio State University, researchers put postretirement-aged rodents into two different social situations. One group lived in a cage that held only two mice—the old-stay-at-home-couple model—while the other group lived in a cage with six mice. After three months, the mice were tested for memory and cognition. The six group-housed mice won hands down. Their brains were working like the brains of healthy young mice. The couple-housed mice not only had decreased memory but also had increased brain inflammation, highly correlated with eroded cognitive health. The brains of the group-housed mice had fewer signs of inflammation, so their brains literally functioned and looked "younger" than the less interactive mice. The part of the brain responsible for memory was physically more robust.

"I've dreamed of group living since my forties," Ceci told me. "It would be fun and practical at the same time. I've always wanted to get a group together to buy a small building in Santa Fe, where I have a strong community. About ten or twelve units, an elevator, obviously. Keep an apartment for younger people to live there and help out with maintenance. We could share resources and caretaking, read, and talk about books and issues to keep each other cognitively in the game. It would be easier for us to spell each other when someone has a partner who's having trouble. It's a built-in support system without being in a nursing home!"

Preservation of cognition is key to the Upgrade, and the people we are bonded with have the greatest impact on long-term cognition than most anything else in our lives. Even the mice are telling us that being stuck at home alone or with only one person can be less stimulating and more damaging to brain function. Inflammation, so present in the brains of the coupled mice, can be responsible for cognitive decline. Keeping our social circles as wide as possible will not only preserve the Upgrade but also help take the pressure off at home.

For better or worse, we master what we repeat. Just as the improving dexterity of a violinist's left hand manifests as increased connectivity in the brain's right motor cortex, women with larger social networks are better at making new social connections. The knock-on effect, according to one study, is that they are less likely to develop dementia than those with smaller networks. Women who had daily contact with friends and family cut their risk of dementia by nearly half. Connection and belonging trigger a soothing cocktail of neurotransmitters that regulate mood and provide a buffer in times of stress and anxiety. Getting together with friends nourishes the brain; girlfriends become the secret weapon of the Upgrade. These interactions may even reset the aging clock.

In a study done in New Hampshire in 1979, psychologist Ellen Langer created a setting for men in their late seventies and early eighties that would bring them back to 1959. The men spent a week in an environment that had Nat King Cole on the radio, newspaper headlines about Castro coming to power in Cuba, brand-new books by Ian Fleming and Leon Uris, and Jackie Gleason on TV. Compared to both a control group that was not immersed in 1959 and to their own results in tests done before they entered the experiment, the men exhibited clear improvements in memory, vision, hearing, and strength. Before and after photos showed that the men looked objectively younger after spending a week together as though it were 1959 instead of 1979. Anything that turns back the aging clock and reduces inflammation is great for the brain. So watch your old childhood favorites on television, listen to and dance to the music of your teen years, and head off to that reunion you've been avoiding. Those old memories are great for resetting the aging clock.

We can reproduce some of the effects of the experiment by consciously activating healthy brain and nervous-system circuits. Visualization is one of the most powerful ways for this to occur, and one of the fastest ways to make change. Try sitting down and taking a few deep breaths, letting your body relax. See if you can remember a moment in your childhood, teen years, or early adulthood when you felt happy, full of fun, at the top of your game. Maybe it was a party, a sleepover, or your first big career boost. Maybe it was the loving excitement your parents showed when you learned a new skill as a child. Spend some time conjuring the details as though you were there right now: the sounds, smells, sights, people, environment, and feelings, both emotions and sensations. Hear the music and feel the laughter. Sense the joy of youthful movement. Let in the deep care for old friends. Take a few minutes and rest in that memory, and notice if there are any changes in your body. It may take a few tries to trick the body into releasing the cascade of feel-good hormones, but it's possible. And if you do this often enough when you're calm, you might have more resilience during tough times, as studies done at Emory University are indicating. I now practice this mental exercise daily and recommend it to my patients.

———

The echoes of old tent-of-"Me" relationship circuits are strong, and not all of us find our way to upgrading them. But we have a choice in the new space that opens in the Upgrade. We can go down the path of despair and worry that comes with the old patterns, with powerlessness over aging, with helplessness over the direction of our children's lives. Or we can stand and make friends with the realities of life. For many of us who value our ability to make things happen, discovering in the Upgrade that there is so much over which we are not in control threatens our sense of competence. But there's so much in store in the Upgrade. We can engage new circuits, shifting our roles in relationships to ones that give us the most freedom to be ourselves. We can feel our own feelings, find our own desires, separate from what's happening for those closest to us. Centering in the Upgrade gives us the space to come to terms with things as they are, to confidently ride the ups and downs instead of fighting them.

Centering

Chapter 10

"So how do you feel about seeing everyone?" I asked my friend Diane, fifty-eight, as she was getting ready for her fortieth high school reunion. Personally, these kinds of gatherings had been my most feared moments of the Transition. I imagined the anxiety Diane must be feeling as the insula (the area of the brain that began torturing us in puberty as we compared ourselves to others and found ourselves lacking) activated memories of social hierarchies, feeling left out if she hadn't been invited to the right party, or not feeling as pretty as the popular girls. I was calling Diane to give a little moral support, making sure she wasn't going through what so many of us do when we are headed into a gathering of people who likely remember us only when our looks were the best they were ever going to be.

When we are teenagers, that high school image of "Me" imprints on the insula as a template for who we are and what we should strive to look like. Its wiring stands at the ready to signal self-disgust when someone shows us a recent photo taken in bright light, when we see ourselves on a video call, when we see the clothes we can no longer wear, when we meet up with a high school friend whom we haven't seen in forty years and think they look younger than we do. Encounters like this can be a perfect nervous-system storm for the female brain, and I was worried that those old tracks in Diane's brain would be prompting a lot of fear and anxiety.

But Diane had an unexpected reaction. "Hey, babe, I'm glad you called, but I am fine," she said. I could hear her rifling through her closet as we spoke, and then the line was silent.

"Diane, honey, you there?" I asked.

"What's this still doing here?" she said quietly. "I thought I tossed it."

"What did you find?"

"It's an old cocktail dress that doesn't fit anymore. I was traumatized by this one," she said. "Remember that phase when you still thought you could beat your changing body into submission?" I remembered all too well. There were a lot of tears involved.

"Back then, I tried to squeeze myself into this dress for my niece's wedding," Diane continued. "My husband hurt his hand trying to zip this one. He knew how badly I wanted to wear it, so he didn't give up. He went out to the garage and got a pair of pliers. He used the pliers to pull the zipper up." Diane started to giggle. "First the little tab on the zipper broke off. Then he managed to get a grip on the zipper itself. He got it zipped, all right; and the whole dress ripped!"

By the time she finished the story, Diane and I were in full-on guffaw. I knew she had been making some changes in her life, but I didn't know she had also been hard at work shifting the neurological and neurochemical tracks in her brain. In particular, she had already laid down new tracks in the insula, tracks that allowed for a sense of "Me" that aligned with her current reality instead of fighting with her "Me" of the past. The insula maps out what is considered beautiful in a culture and then engages in constant comparison. Diane had upgraded from the teenaged Insula 18.0 to Insula 58.0. She was staying healthy, eating well, and exercising, and she wasn't setting unrealistic goals, like trying to fight her way down to the weight she was at eighteen. She had come to terms with a larger midsection, crow's-feet, lip lines, a wrinkled neck, and a little bit of jowl. She had decided life was too short to feel bad about her neck.

"It took me a while to get to this place," she said when I asked about how she was managing the Upgrade. "That scene wasn't funny at the time. I tried on two more dresses, and none of them fit. I was sobbing and I had black lines streaming down my face. An hour of work on hair and makeup was down the drain. I love my niece and we are very close, but by the time I squeezed into a third dress, I didn't want to go to the wedding. My husband was amazing. I was falling apart, and he was comforting and persistent. He knew I'd regret it for the rest of my life if I didn't get myself there. I finally found something loose and black—I know, you're not supposed to wear black to a wedding, but it was that or yoga pants. We arrived an hour late; I missed the ceremony altogether, and I didn't know what to tell my sister. I got as close to the truth as I could and told them that I had been sick. I guess after they read this they'll know what really happened!"

"Oh, honey," I said, "I've been there. I remember those battles." I had many in my fifties, in the Early Upgrade. Listening to Diane, I could feel the creeping sense of disgust at myself, echoes of my own Insula 18.0. The battle with the body and the shift to embracing a new reality is a developmental phase in the Early and Middle Upgrade, one that we don't talk about.

Like Ceci, Diane had decided to give away everything that didn't fit and look for a style that made her feel comfortable now. "I had to get rid of the reminders," she said, "for the sake of my own mental health, and my husband's poor fingers."

Diane's action made sense from an Upgrade perspective. If she was opening a closet twice a day to a rack full of clothes that didn't fit, she was activating the insula in its task of comparison, which all too easily escalates into self-blame and self-flagellation. Those attitudes signal the pituitary to send out a hormone prompting the adrenals to open a fire hose of distress hormones. Those hormones trigger the brain and nervous system to cause jitters, anxiety, and testiness. If we allow those old neurological tracks to take over, hopelessness, even intractable melancholy, can be the outcome. In those with diagnosed depression, that pituitary signal to the adrenals is already stuck on high, and stress hormones pour out nonstop. Not everyone can cope without medication, but many of us, like Diane, are not helpless. Developing strategies for shifting the tracks of Insula

18.0 was an important step in upgrading the insula to align with Diane's sense of the tent of "Me" at fifty-eight.

"I thought my closet was cleaned out," she said, "but this one must have escaped. It's going to Goodwill first thing tomorrow!"

So many patients and friends have reported that during the Transition and in their Early Upgrade, issues they thought they'd dealt with re-emerge, hijacking the nervous system with unexpected force. The energy to muscle through is gone.

It can be triggered by something as small as someone disagreeing with our opinion or leaving us out; it can be a time when the world no longer responds to who we believe we are. It can happen when we encounter a reminder of an old trauma. Every day, and more so as we enter the Transition and the Upgrade, life circumstances, old wounds, and people's reactions to us challenge our tent of "Me." It happens even to the strongest of us, those who went through years of therapy and lots of hard work to address issues large and small. It happens as we become fed up with old caretaking roles, only to find ourselves sucked back into them. And as I can attest, it happens a decade after we negotiated peace with our body, when we think we long ago ended the lifetime of war. It happens when we find ourselves taking on extra work for free because someone managed to find and push our "good girl" button and we jumped to volunteer. It happens when we realize those occupying the space closest to our tent pole may have wrested control right out of our hands (or we voluntarily handed the control over once again), throwing our sense of priorities into disarray.

Waves leave imprints. Wading through calm waters, we feel their ridges in the sand beneath our feet, evidence of their passage. Though our hormonal waves may have calmed in the Upgrade, their echoes are still imprinted in the tent of "Me." In certain situations, echoes can become amplified, activating tracks that were laid in another time, reminders that push our neurohormonal (and emotional) buttons, pulling us off balance, sending us spiraling out of healthy self-care into sadness, fear, isolation—"I didn't want to go to the wedding"—and sometimes self-loathing.

Becoming centered is a gift of the Upgrade; yet unrecognized echoes of the old waves threaten our ability to manifest that gift. Those old patterns of who we thought we were as a woman in her fertility phase—how we should look, feel, socialize, exercise, eat, engage in care of others and ourselves—can pull us out of our zone of well-being faster than you can say "hot flash." To emerge into an optimized Upgrade means using our attention and our intelligence to take full control of our own tent pole, learning how to keep it from being yanked out of the ground or snapped in half by echoes of waves that no longer pound the shores. It means being able to remain still even as the echoes of old hurts, old wounds, try to pull us off center. Hitting an obstacle doesn't throw you off your horse anymore. When something is emotionally upsetting, you realize that if you put one foot in front of the other, within forty-eight to seventy-two hours the sting reduces on its own. We develop the strength of holding the space to see what happens, resisting the impulse to act. As those waves weaken, we can watch them dissolve into a warm, gentle foam as we wade more easily along the shore where we once sat and brooded.

Tina Sloan is an actress who played the role of nurse Lillian Raines on *Guiding Light* for twenty-six years. In her book *Changing Shoes: Getting Older—NOT OLD—with Style, Humor, and Grace,* she talks about the day she experienced the *coup de vieux,* the "blow of age." On a break from shooting a party scene, she and her on-screen daughter headed out for coffee in ball gowns. As a soap opera star who had been counseled as a teenager by the cream of French society on how to command a room and the attention of men, she was used to wielding that power. But on this day, in this café in Midtown Manhattan, at nearly fifty years old, she could feel something was off. It was unsettling, and she wasn't sure what it was. And then she realized that the attention of the men in the café was riveted by her costar, not her. She felt disoriented as the tent of "Me" she was accustomed to experiencing felt like it was being blown away.

It was the insula noticing something was off-kilter as her nervous system waited for the familiar stares of admiration. When those signals did not come, her memory circuits set off the alarm: *We are not in balance.* In parallel, the vagal system—the body and brain's largest nerve, responsible for both activating and calming the body's threat system—picked up the alert. Acting as a superhighway among the intestines, the heart, and the brain, the vagus triggered a literal gut instinct that something was wrong. The nerves were begging her brain, *Do something to get us back to our cushion of familiarity at the center of the tent of "Me."*

The push to *do something* comes in the form of brain signals to produce neurohormones that drive behavior. There are so many responses that can satiate the hunger for a familiar response, and the responses we choose can be determined by whether or not we've been able to upgrade the insula. If we are slaving under the oppression of Insula 18.0, then the signals can be torture. Accustomed to being recognized as the hot one, when a hotter one comes on the scene, the insula sends out a red alert that you're not going to get the good sperm. It flashes *insufficient* to your sense of self, sending a hot poker to your nervous system to make your prefrontal cortex start doing its job of problem solving. Even though those old fertility hormones might be gone, the echoes of them can create a flurry of activity. I've seen those urges manifest in friends, patients, and myself when Insula 18.0 rips at the tent pole and stability of our sense of "Me."

Resisting the impulse to react to the insula's commands barked at the prefrontal cortex is hard, but finding a way to take our foot off the gas is a quality-of-life decision. When Jacqueline de La Chaume moved from Paris to the United States with her husband, Yul Brynner, she was warned by her old friend, Karl Lagerfeld, not to give in to cosmetic-procedure pressure in Hollywood. And she said that Yul was against it as well, telling her that it would erase the map of her life as it appeared on her face. The pressure can feel real. I've made and canceled appointments for procedures dozens of times myself.

"It's hard to watch what's going on among the women here," Sarah said after moving to Houston. "You see women in their late eighties not eating, wobbling around in high heels, wigs, and heavy makeup. Their cheeks and lips are stuffed full of fillers. Many in my generation—in our fifties—just aren't doing this anymore. There's something tragic about seeing women being pulled away from themselves like this, unable to express who they really are." Sarah is right. Statistics are showing that those getting cosmetic procedures are skewing younger, to the before-the-Transition years. It's too soon to tell if women in the Early Upgrade aren't getting the procedures because they already did them in their thirties and forties or if this is a real trend away from cosmetic procedures.

When we become centered, able to remain grounded in order to honor the woman who's emerging, the neurological mindset shift of the Upgrade frees us from the struggle to prolong the appearance of the fertility phase. Although these decisions are very personal and I don't feel it's right to judge, I do admire Tina Sloan's choice as an actress never to have her face altered by cosmetic procedures. It tells me that she made a decision to take control of her own tent pole, her visceral sense of who she is.

When it comes to appearance in the Upgrade, what I'm talking about goes beyond acceptance to loving engagement and unconditional embrace. A begrudging stance toward ourselves is still destructive, like continuing to sneak nourishment to Insula 18.0 even as we are trying to shape the tent of "Me" 2.0. As our peer group makes different decisions—some opting for an Upgrade, others opting to go to war against nature, friendships shift.

What We Are Up Against

Female fertility is at the core of our social fabric. As children we played house and perhaps fought over who got to play the mommy. We bonded secretly over the beginning of our periods and our first sexual encounters. Many of us built our own families; around our kids another social life formed as we got to know the parents of their friends at school. Those of us without children formed bonds at work and through volunteering. Disruption first comes if you are divorced, and possibly shut out by married girlfriends, or are aged out of a job and career. And when the kids grow up and leave, the social bonds formed around them and the roles we've played are also gone.

As older women we are marginalized, dehumanized, labeled as cute, called "young lady" or "a little holiday angel of cheer," as two young women in Atlanta addressed fifty-four-year-old Terri one time while she was dropping off her dry cleaning. If we have allowed the nervous system to absorb that narrative, then it amplifies the signal that we are not relevant. It indicates that we should stop caring for ourselves and paves the path to social isolation. This doesn't become garden-variety loneliness; the nervous system begins to lose the ability to engage the circuitry that keeps us reaching out to connect, to keep those essential brain vitamins we receive through community that nurture the desire to keep putting one foot in front of the other every day. This is likely an underlying contributor to the alarming rise in suicide among women over sixty. Twenty-five percent of women will have a major clinical depression sometime in their life. If you've had a major melancholic episode before the transition, it means that you are two to three times more likely to have another one post-Transition. If we absorb the message that we don't matter, melancholy is often a consequence. How we feel about how the world sees us can make the Upgrade challenging.

I was listening to NPR one Friday morning in early March of 2020 when I heard about a United Nations Development Programme (UNDP) report about attitudes toward women. The study was conducted across seventy-five countries, and the report concluded that nearly 90 percent of all human beings are biased against women at work, in government, for their opinions, in every area of life. I had two reactions. First I thought, *Did I hear that right? Ninety percent?* I called a friend, who found the *Guardian* story on the report. Indeed, I had heard it right.

Deep down I wasn't surprised by this news. The bigger surprise was that this massive obstacle to feeling free to claim our common human dignity, to stand firmly in the experience that our rights and needs are equal to others', was finally being reported on.

And then the harder truth hit me square in the face. The report didn't find that 90 percent of men were biased against women; the finding indicated that on average, nearly 90 percent of all human beings are biased against women, and that 86 percent of women were biased against women. It made me question who was in the 14 percent; I suddenly had to consider that if women were biased against their own gender, then there were likely men in that tiny group of allies who weren't. I also had to face that I might be part of that 86 percent of women who engage in hostile sexism toward my own gender.

In my psychiatric training I learned about the concept of introjection, when an individual absorbs the perspective of another or their culture and makes it part of themselves. It is particularly common in anyone in a weaker position who feels the need to agree with the stronger one in order to survive. I knew that at various points, especially in my twenties, I had introjected some form of hostile sexism. It happens unconsciously during the epoch of competition for the best sperm. No matter how feminist we are, the hormones coursing through our bodies during the fertility phase ping the brain continuously to drive actions and behaviors dedicated to optimizing procreation. As young women dominated by neurohormones, we often turned away from anything we perceived as being distasteful to men. If younger men derided sexism and feminism, we often did too. I remember sometimes feeling that women's groups were stupid; I was convinced older women were just jealous of us because they had lost their hotness. That I feel the opposite now is not just about education, experience, and the fact that I am now an older woman. It has a lot to do with the easing of neurohormones that drove those earlier attitudes. In the Upgrade, this is another bias that can drop away.

New Source of Validation

Many of us talk about having been much more disciplined in our younger lives about taking care of ourselves, and that post-Transition our efforts feel intermittent, scattered, uneven. The signals we got to take care of ourselves when we were younger were, no matter how enlightened we thought we were, driven by fertility hormones and cultural messages about showing off our health and ability to procreate. It was important to the survival of the species that we be healthy when young; cultural obsession with youth and beauty is really just a symptom. It's not a coincidence that in the second half we have a harder time focusing and maintaining our efforts—we don't feel society's deep care about our health. It can feel harder to remember which tools to use or which people to call who have helped us emerge from problems in the past. The signals we get after the Transition about our importance to the culture at large are devastating: that once we lose our eggs, we don't matter; that we should give up, especially since nearly everybody we encounter in a single day is biased against us as women. Though the UNDP report didn't break out bias by age, it is reasonable to conjecture that for women over the age of forty-five or fifty, the experience of bias could easily climb higher.

Every decision takes bandwidth. We have the opportunity to choose how much bandwidth we want to expend on diet plans, hair color, dermatologists, and makeup. Some of those decisions didn't feel optional during the fertility phase. But now they might be. "I am wearing the same stretchy shirts and pants," Ceci said. "And in my world, being chic was very important. I paid a lot of attention to it, shopped in Italy, and treated my clothes like an investment portfolio. But at a certain point I realized it was such a big waste of time and money," she continued. "Now I have the same freedom I had when I wore a uniform in high school. It wasn't restrictive. It was freeing. I didn't have to decide what to wear." In her Upgrade, Katharine Hepburn wore black pants and a white collared shirt every day for the last thirty years of her life. Jacqueline de La Chaume, who in the 1960s worked for designer André Courrèges and for *Vogue Paris,* began making her own simple clothes in her sixties. In my sixties, I choose athleisure. I can free up my nervous system's bandwidth by not stressing over a decision that no longer feels important to me.

Many women in the Upgrade found this freedom in the lockdown during the COVID-19 pandemic, when we suddenly saw how much energy was dedicated to purely fabricated standards around appearance. Now we know that without contact with others, we wear whatever we want. The deep relief many felt is a window on what it would be like to make that choice under normal circumstances.

When we are no longer trying to have it all, when we recognize that there are real limits to what can be accomplished and we can accept them, we can be free of the torture of unrealistic goals remaining constantly out of reach. We can see freedom in the Upgrade instead of lack.

We can shift from mourning the loss of fertility to enjoying the freedom of not having to freak out about pregnancy, mood swings, blood, or cramps. We can enjoy the freedom of walking down the street without the burden of the voracious stares of men, the whistling, the catcalls. We can enjoy that drugstore shopping time is cut because there is an entire aisle we never have to walk down again—unless our daughter-in-law or granddaughter is visiting.

Remember, biology is destiny if you don't know what it's doing to you. By recognizing the biological and neurochemical principles in the female brain, we can see which circuits we are reinforcing through our physical, mental, and emotional habits. Becoming mindful and alert means we have a unique opportunity to reshape the circuits during this time. The Upgrade supports us in this endeavor. And if we are lucky, the internal voice of the centering circuits can become so strong that they are no longer suggestible to old habits. The tent pole becomes unshakable. And what you decide to do with your tent matters to me.

Body Hacks for the Mind

Chapter 11

Let's say I went to sleep angry about something that happened with my husband, my son, or a friend. I'm in a fitful state most of the night, not really resting. I wake up thinking about the argument, replaying it in my head, rehearsing the words I wish I'd been quick enough to think of, willing a different outcome with all my might, priming myself for more anger and probably another argument.

The mind serves up all kinds of thoughts during the night in the form of dreams, and more when we wake up. This is completely normal. Sometimes a whole scene from the past, something that is very upsetting, will arise full blown and hijack my thinking circuits. Trying to block or suppress the thoughts or memories that make us uncomfortable doesn't work—they tend to come back in another form and sometimes even stronger. While we are busy trying to keep old anger from surfacing, we might take it out on someone nearby.

The biggest biological impact on emotion is hormones. Hormones drive behavior. Ghrelin makes us want to eat. Testosterone makes us want to have sex. Oxytocin makes us want to repair a relationship. Progesterone makes us want to curl up under a blanket. Cortisol and adrenaline, the stress hormones set off by frustration, danger, fear, or anger, can make us want to lash out to protect ourselves.

A burst of cortisol, say from a big argument, can continue affecting the body and brain for many hours—assuming there isn't another stressor to set off another round of it. Then it can take up to five days for the brain to reset to the new normal and for access to circuits of higher reason and judgment to become fully accessible again. And in the Upgrade, the effects of cortisol can be prolonged, especially if you have a stressed partner. So that old adage about cooling off for twenty-four hours before responding to a highly charged situation? It isn't nearly long enough. A week and a day is more like it. If we try to respond or to problem-solve while we are at the mercy of our hormones, we are more likely to develop what psychologists call emotional incontinence. We just can't hold it in; we can't contain the extremes of emotion, so we cross a line with words or the slam of a door. Escalation increases stress and the cortisol cycle starts all over again.

Cortisol, the classic stress hormone, naturally rises early in the morning to help us wake up, raise our blood pressure, and achieve alertness, getting us ready to learn new things and be at the top of our mental game. It also rises when we perceive a threat of any kind, from an irritating news story to a narrowly avoided car accident. Levels can rise with aging and be higher in older females than in older males. But chronic rumination or intractable melancholy can intensify cortisol, making levels high enough to disable clear thinking and problem-solving altogether. It can also set off a chain reaction that causes sterile inflammation of tissues and blood vessels, even in the brain. Add to that lower estrogen, which in our earlier days protected cognition against stress, and we can be set up for a more rapid mental decline. Even if we are taking HT, chronic stress and rumination can run roughshod over estrogen's protective benefits. Stress can be one of the most dangerous enemies to cognition in the second half.

As a doctor who specializes in the brain, of course I prioritize its health. It's a natural bias when you love something as much as I love the female brain. But there's also deep justification. Strong and healthy cognition is key to being able to manifest the best qualities of the female brain in the Upgrade. When we make choices that hinder the brain's capacity to remain strong, vibrant, and sharp, we can all too easily slip into smaller and sadder worlds that can spiral into isolation and melancholy. In my practice over the decades, I've seen this happen too many times, watched too many women slip into a preventable downgrade. But simple changes—even changes as simple as moving your body—play a huge role in preserving cognition, especially in the face of stress.

Movement Is Cognition; Cognition Is Movement

My patient Rhonda, sixty-eight, is a social worker. Super comfortable with her age, she let her hair go white in her early sixties. It took ten years off her face and helped revive her part-time acting career: She was able to land a few small parts in some big films. In that regard, she shifted her tent of "Me" to incorporate her changing physical identity. She also decided never to have any cosmetic procedures on her face.

Rhonda takes her Upgrade seriously. She is a gregarious and outgoing woman, a friendly and generous person—until a younger woman or man dares to "young lady" or "dear" her. "It started happening in my fifties," she told me. "I won't answer when someone asks, 'And how are we today, young lady?' But if they persist, I have my response cued up: 'I hope you aren't addressing me. I haven't been called *young lady* since I was five and in trouble with my mother. I am a grown woman. I am proud of every single year and every single wrinkle. You can call me *ma'am*. No, not *dear*. Ma'am.'"

Rhonda had been working out regularly, taking yoga, strength training, and going on long, fast walks for cardio conditioning. When she feels physically strong, her confidence rises and she feels able to stay centered in the face of slights and difficulties. But life has many blows to deliver.

After a long period of stability, Rhonda's thirty-four-year-old daughter Seana, who suffers from bipolar disease, went off her meds and off the rails. Seana walked out on her husband and four-year-old daughter and took up residence on the streets of LA, trading sex for drugs, as she had done in her teen years. After a few weeks Seana disappeared from the neighborhood and Rhonda had no way of finding her daughter. Rhonda became despondent, listless, unable to think or express herself clearly. Her tent of "Me" as a mother was in collapse. As a social worker, she knew intellectually that her daughter's disease was not her fault and was not within her control to cure. But as a mother, she turned every drop of guilt she could find into a psychological bat with which to beat herself. It didn't change her outward circumstances or help her find her daughter, but it intensified her stress and sorrow.

In times of profound chronic stress, the cortisol-releasing hormone CRH can get stuck on high, eventually depleting the system and its circuitry of the fuels that might otherwise motivate us to get up and move. It's like running an engine at its highest RPM, burning out the motor to the point that it seizes up. Now scientists believe that when people get profound melancholic depression, and in particular melancholic depression post-Transition, it affects their movement system. In these extreme cases patients report feeling stuck curled in the fetal position. We used to think the will to move was all that was missing. Now we know that the motor system also goes into a clinical depression along with motivation and mood. This is why, as a psychiatrist, after I've tried everything else, I now recommend taking an integrated mind-body approach to profound sadness.

Rhonda was an old patient of mine for whom antidepressants had terrible side effects. When her husband, Mike, called concerned about Rhonda's state of mind, I knew drugs wouldn't be an option. But new information about a brain organ called the cerebellum was opening the door to a different way to help.

Many times, when babies start to crawl, they will pull themselves along the floor using only their arms, dragging the lower part of the body behind them. Getting their knees underneath them, coordinating their alternating movements—right arm, left leg, left arm, right leg—is the job of the headband-shaped motor cortex, which wraps around the top of the brain and communicates down to the coordinator of motion, the cerebellum. But different systems of the brain turn on at different times during the first year of life, and sometimes nature needs a little help from Mom and Dad. This is often a simple fix: With your baby lying on her back, make a game of holding her feet and bicycling her legs. Then help her stand and hold her hands while she stomps her feet. Feeling and watching the movement sends a signal backward from the eyes and muscles via the nerves to the cerebellum: *Hey up there! Start your engine for this part of the body. I need to move!* It's not usually very long before the wiring develops a strong and steady signal that kicks the cerebellum into gear to organize the signals sent by the motor cortex. Baby is off and running, and you are getting more exercise than you planned chasing after her.

When Mike got Rhonda to agree to a phone consultation, I decided to test a thought that we could do something similar for her, using movement to trigger emotional stability. "Rhonda, can you put me on video and set the phone down?" I asked her during our first call. Knowing that she had practiced yoga since her twenties, I took a chance on her muscle memory. She placed the phone on a table and I asked her to stand nearby. "Now, feel your feet on the ground. Feel the sensation of contact on the bottoms of your feet. Close your eyes and let your attention rest there for a bit."

"Oh my goodness, my legs are shaking!"

"I know," I responded. This can happen as attention signals nerves to fire, as in Rhonda's case, to make her legs feel stronger than she felt emotionally. "Don't worry about it. Just let them shake. Feel your feet."

"Okay," she said after a silence. "They stopped. I'm ready. What's next?"

"Make sure your feet are hip distance apart. Now settle there, and when you are comfortable, slowly shift your weight to one side."

"That feels really unsteady. I feel like I might fall."

"Okay, open your eyes a little. Don't focus on anything. Let your attention drop to the foot you have your weight on. Tell me when you feel comfortable. Don't rush."

"Okay. I'm okay."

"Now lift the other foot. Stay there for a while. Get your balance. Focus on a spot on the floor and breathe for a few counts. Feel the sole of the standing foot. Then gently put the lifted foot down again; feel the sensation of contact with the floor. When you are ready, shift to the other side and lift the other foot." We did this a few times until Rhonda could maintain her balance on one foot with some reliability. When her physical balance began to stabilize, I started to hear a tiny bit of light in Rhonda's voice. When she lifted the phone again, I could see her face had begun to relax.

"Okay, this is great, Rhonda," I said. "Now let's try a little more movement. Is it nice outside?"

"It's cloudy," she said, "but it's okay to go outside."

"Can you plug in your headphones and put the phone in your pocket?" I asked.

"Yes, sure."

"Okay, let's go, then. I just want you to walk slowly, deliberately, paying attention to each step to the end of the block and back."

"That's it?"

"Yes, that's it." I remained silent on the phone. Rhonda reported feeling unsteady and off balance. I kept suggesting she return her attention to the soles of her feet, feeling the movement of her legs, finding balance by noticing that spot in the center of the body behind the navel, the center of gravity for the female body.

"Boy, this is starting to feel good," she said after a few minutes. "But my legs feel a little shaky at this slow pace. I can't balance when the anxiety starts to come up again."

"Yes, that's normal. So breathe slowly, walk deliberately," I reminded her. "And let's try it again."

As Rhonda moved, her pronunciation became clearer and her words came more easily. Her voice relaxed and sounded less constricted. Movement began to impact Rhonda's mood and her cognition.

I asked her to practice alternate-nostril breathing (see appendix, page 258) and a balancing exercise every day, followed by a very slow brief walk. As she became steadier, I suggested she try walking mindfully along a seam in her wood floor as though it were a tightrope. Over time, Rhonda's clarity began to return. Mike confirmed that Rhonda had become much calmer and was beginning to return to her old talkative self again.

Old Wounds, New Approach

Deep in the back, at the bottom of the brain, hanging near the base of the skull like two big ovaries, is the cerebellum. For more than one hundred years, neurologists and neuroscientists have known that the cerebellum is a command center for movement, balance, and fine motor skills. When combined with visual and inner-ear input, it is responsible for how we learn new dance steps and drills in soccer, how we know where to put our feet as we watch where we are walking or running. With the addition of a mirror, the cerebellum helps us perfect positions in yoga or ballet. It's one of the oldest parts of the brain; it's present in our reptile and aquatic cousins, helping fish orient their movement in the undulations of the sea.

The cerebellum is super sensitive to alcohol, and it's why, after a few glasses of wine, we might drive erratically and have a tough time maintaining balance on that straight line on which the officer asks us to walk. If we are nervous or very upset, the cerebellum is inhibited by the body's threat response; right after we receive very bad news, the flood of cortisol and other adrenal neurohormones makes it more likely we will bump into things, break things, or crash our cars. If the cerebellum is injured, we will have a hard time buttoning our clothing or guiding a spoonful of oatmeal to our mouths.

Most fMRIs that study the brain's functioning and connectivity easily image the brain areas above the cerebellum, like the frontal cortex, the visual cortex, the parietal cortex, the amygdala, and other brain organs. We are, as a result, more familiar with the blood flow and connectedness of these areas of problem-solving, interpreting visual stimuli, processing sensory information, and initiating muscle movement, and the brain's center of fear. Because of its location so deep and below the brain's big hemispheres, it's been tougher to get a clear picture of the cerebellum and study its connectivity to other parts of the brain. For the better part of the last century, neuroscientists felt the role and responsibility of the cerebellum for coordinating motion and balance was settled, so it remained ignored in the basement of the brain.

But in 2018 we got a big surprise. One of the very few labs in the world that has the capacity to image the cerebellum via a special functional MRI was able to see that its connectivity to other parts of the brain was dramatically more complex than anyone had imagined. Scientists at Washington University in St. Louis discovered that motor coordination was only one-fifth of the cerebellum's job. By observing connectivity to other parts of the brain, they learned that 80 percent of the cerebellum's functioning was related to areas that deal with judgment, problem-solving and the ability to think in the abstract, emotion and mood, memory, and language. The cerebellum, the hub of movement, balance, and coordination, is involved in editing almost everything we ask our brain to do. It fine-tunes emotional and cognitive function just the way it fine-tunes muscle movement. It makes learning and social engagement possible. It's a key to motivation, that feeling of being psyched up. It's only 10 percent of the brain's volume, but it holds more than 50 percent of the brain's neurons (brain/nerve cells).

Just as estrogen stimulates the prefrontal cortex (PFC), boosting our mental acuity and access to the problem-solving functions of the brain, progesterone helps boost functionality in the cerebellum. When it functions optimally, the cerebellum is a kind of filter, checking thoughts, emotions, and sensory information for spam, phishing, or scams before letting you act on or express them. As the original researchers point out, the cerebellum doesn't think, balance, or judge; it corrects errors and helps the parts of the brain that are responsible for those activities do their job more efficiently. A healthy cerebellum will check impulses as they emerge to make sure acting on them is good for your ability to thrive. If it's not a good idea, the cerebellum will delete it. If it is a good idea, the cerebellum will help recruit brain and nervous system resources to express it and act upon it. If it's impaired by alcohol, it won't be able to stop us from speaking or acting impulsively. Drunk driving and drunk texting both emanate from the same source.

Psychologists and researchers have long known that when it comes to sadness and clinical depression, aerobic exercise is at least as effective as antidepressants in making a productive shift. The new information on the cerebellum tells us much more about how this might work. Because it is connected to the emotion, reward, and judgment centers of the brain, physical and emotional balance can be understood as part of the same process, part of the same drive for overall homeostasis.

Homeostasis is the dynamic balance that every living system strives for in its mission to optimize survival. It's not a static state; it's a process of unending microadjustments made to approximate some mythical permanent state of well-being. Like the ballast correcting a sailboat's angle in a strong wind, the cerebellum helps us push back against what throws us off, both physically and emotionally. When physical balance is upset, the cerebellum triggers movement-stabilizing circuits, fine-tuning them so that we stand or sit firmly upright again. When emotional balance is upset, we can enlist muscle movement to help bring the cerebellum's capacity back online—practicing physical balance can help with melancholy, for example. And in some cases we might be able to jump-start the engine of stability by combining attention and movement, as Rhonda did.

This new way of understanding the cerebellum has led me to include it in my evaluations of patients, especially those who are falling more often. If Rhonda, for example, had not been able to regain her physical balance, and if she had been falling more than normal, after getting a brain MRI, I might have started to look for decline in cognition, for lapses in judgment. If the cerebellum is not able to coordinate movement and balance, it is likely having trouble coordinating language, emotion regulation, and stress response.

These days I don't just prescribe meds for profound sadness. For those who need the support, I definitely still do write prescriptions. But I also prescribe a gentle ten-to-twenty-minute walk once a day, a walking meditation, a gratefulness or prayer walk, extending the time gradually to an hour if it's possible. It doesn't cure everything, but it helps bring feelings of sadness into a manageable range, so that we can apply other strategies to regain control of our tent pole. Being able to restart our habit of self-care determines our resilience in the face of the difficulties we know are bound to come.

It took about two months for Rhonda to restart her fitness routine. "I'm still utterly anxious and worried over Seana," she told me. She'd since gotten news that her daughter had been found and had agreed to go into a treatment facility. It was a relief, but Rhonda had been here many times before, and she was still quite worried over whether or not this round would stick for Seana. It's normal to be in a fearful state when times are tough, either personally or globally, to have anxiety levels that remain at a persistent five out of ten. But we have a chance to change things once the hormonal spikes of the Transition have evened out. We can use that new steadiness to introduce a few tricks for nudging the brain's system for clarity and calm.

Cultivating Joy

"I was running five miles three times a week, and on the weekend I often did back-to-back classes at the gym," Sarah, forty-eight, told me. "I'd been doing this for years, and it was magical. I was tiny, eating healthy mostly but knowing if I cheated I could just burn it off. Regular, intense exercise every morning before work made me sleep better at night for a long time. But when I hit the Transition, I went through an insomnia nightmare. I kept waking up at three and couldn't go back to sleep. It felt like I couldn't handle the stress of work anymore. I lost the certainty I had when I was in my thirties and started second-guessing myself all the time. I couldn't absorb the normal ups and downs of life. I couldn't sleep if I watched the news past eight P.M. I couldn't sleep if my husband mentioned money at ten P.M. Working out had been my go-to stress reducer and my most reliable weight-control plan. And when I hit the Transition and it got, well, a bit spectacular, with bleeding and irregularity, I got devastating advice from my doctor: Rest. Do yoga. Stop running. Meditate. Take gentle walks. Sit on a park bench and look at the river. I had never sat still!"

I knew just what she meant and why that prescription felt devastating. Sarah continued, "I had no choice but to follow directions, because I didn't have the energy to keep up my old pace anymore. I was terrified I would start to feel sad because I couldn't kick up the endorphin high of running. I was terrified of becoming depressed if my weight ballooned. And it did. I gained twenty-five pounds in one year."

Sarah went into a tailspin, canceling social events and refusing to travel to her close friend Kim's fiftieth birthday party, putting the relationship at risk. "My moods were so unpredictable, I couldn't fit into my wardrobe, and I couldn't bear for anyone to see me like this. I tried to explain to Kim that I didn't want to ruin her big day by being so depressed at such a happy occasion, but she said I was ruining it by not coming. She didn't talk to me for a year."

Lack of sleep, feelings of uncertainty, and torture by self-image constantly trigger our threat systems, causing cortisol spikes that make us lash out and pack on the pounds. Grief over the loss of everything that comes with fertility—energy, appearance, attention, vibrance—sets in, and the sense of who we are begins to destabilize. Insula 18.0 had struck again.

The Transition can overwhelm the mind with deep insecurity as the sense of who we are seems to unravel. The longer we are subject to excess chronic cortisol and adrenaline, the more they alter our perception of the motives of others. Seeing threats and insults everywhere, we retreat from connection, and in isolation, the stress cocktail kicks off negative rumination. On the other hand, playful acceptance stimulates joy and optimism; optimism is another key to cognitive health and can be protective against dying from cardiovascular issues.

"We are not going to talk it out," Sarah's husband, Dan, said one night. She was spiraling into hypercriticism over everything and everyone at their book club. Her perception of others' negativity was interfering with their ability to socialize as a couple and sparking huge fights. Dan was determined to break the cycle, and the pressure made him creative. He had passed through the living room one day while she was watching Grey's Anatomy. The two main characters had been talking about their problems, and they started dancing instead of continuing the conversation. "Get up," he said. "We are not going to talk this out. We are going to dance it out." Sarah felt completely foolish, and at first she couldn't get into it. Part of it was the age difference; Dan was thirteen years older, and the music he was playing didn't resonate with her junior high school dance years. Once he switched from the Beatles to Earth, Wind & Fire, Sarah couldn't help herself. She had to move. "I couldn't stop smiling," she said. "I forgot why I was so upset."

Movement is connected to our first success at survival as babies. We reach for the breast and get it. We grab a piece of food from the table and guide it toward our mouths. The reward system for movement is enormous because survival depends on it. We reach, grab, practice, master. *I got that sucker. Yay! I will live.* The basic neuromuscular circuitry of survival rewards us with feelings of success.

The expression of joy is hardwired to muscle movement. Throw your arms up and out to the sides and it begins to stimulate the process, or strike a power pose, the superhero stance that is proven to stimulate confidence and lift the mood through the neuromuscular feedback loop. Add music to movement and the entire nervous system is recruited, bypassing cognition, igniting the heart, circulation, and breathing. I like to blast "Start Me Up" by the Rolling Stones and dance like crazy on my deck, throwing my arms up with almost every beat.

Play is commingled with joy in the nervous system, and before you tell me you've outgrown the need, I'm going to let science set you straight: It's one of our oldest evolutionary instincts, and its impact on cognition is profound. Play is a key nutrient for cognition and the Upgrade. The neurobiology of play impacts key circuitry essential to social skills, creativity, adaptability, problem-solving, and raw intelligence. Scientists have found that the inability to play is a sign of lack of healthy social interactions in rats, and of psychiatric disorder in humans.

Age can determine how much play we need, but not the way you might think it does. We need it most during tough times or after periods of isolation—think post-COVID-lockdown-years—and that need can be more frequent in adulthood, as there is often more to be stressed about. In difficult times, whether personal or societal, we need to play more than ever; it's the very means by which we prepare for the unexpected, search out new solutions, and remain optimistic. It's key circuitry for the brain's hopefulness.

Joy feeds back hopefulness into the nervous system, and hope is pure heroin to the brain. Triggering dopamine to course through the system, it's a massive stimulus to cognition. It ignites creativity and problem-solving, and it becomes contagious in our relationships. The familiar banter among girlfriends that can make you laugh so hard you cry or pee a little, collaborative efforts like working a puzzle with family, or trivia games with friends, stimulate the release of all kinds of feel-good neuro-chemicals.

We can bring a playful attitude to all physical activity. Instead of barking orders at the body, try asking permission, making sure you have consensus from body parts, muscles, and the nervous system. At the beginning of my swim class, I smile at all the parts that make me move and say, "Come on girls, let's jump in!" That lets me start the class with joy. It helps me benefit even more from the exercise and deepen my connection to myself. I become more attuned and aligned. If you can deepen that connection, you not only find new energy, focus, and efficiency but also have a wider bandwidth for others. You can start having fun with yourself and even smile at everyone's foibles.

Drink a shot of joy every day by moving to music, walking in nature, jumping into a pool. Do something playful and something challenging or new every day. Take up space. When you go to the gym, occupy the weight room. Like the warrior stance, it tells the brain that you are powerful. Just don't let exuberance override your better judgment about how much you can lift.

When the Joy Circuits Need a Jump Start

Movement and play don't work for everyone, and they might not work for those with clinically diagnosed issues. Intractable melancholy is a risk for women in the second half of life; if you've had an episode before the Transition, your risk is increased of having another one after.

In the face of threat, the brain's amygdala kicks the hypothalamus to send out corticotrophin-releasing hormone (CRH) to the pituitary, and that signals it to release ACTH (adrenocorticotropic hormone), which gets the puppy-dog adrenals to release cortisol and adrenaline. It's been well known for over thirty years that CRH gets stuck on high in clinical depression. Instead of the usual waves of adrenal cortisol that wake you in the morning, and the drop at 3:00 P.M. that helps you wind down for the day, CRH turns the adrenals into a nonstop cortisol firehose. The body's adrenaline keeps you running like you're taking diet pills or speed. You become hyperfocused, and negative rumination spins out of control day and night. You don't want to eat and you can't sleep. It's a recipe for intractable melancholy. If the rumination spiral becomes fueled by pessimism, it can impact cognition. When you throw in the estrogen spikes and plunges of the Transition, it scrambles the brain completely.

For many women in the Transition, adding estrogen and progesterone can soften the wildness of the waves by calming the brain's spiky demands for a dwindling supply in the ovaries. But since the Women's Health Initiative (WHI) report, doctors have started to increase the amount of SSRIs (selective serotonin reuptake inhibitors) they are prescribing for mood and hot flashes instead of hormones. (See appendix, page 257.) SSRIs work predictably for mood and hot flashes in only about 30 to 60 percent of women. I have had some women respond nicely, but there is a chance they won't work well for you. In addition, no one has ever done a proper long-term study on how these drugs interact with the Transition.

Over the course of my thirty years at the UCSF clinic, by the time a woman in the Transition would come to see me, she would be at the end of her rope emotionally. She had usually already been through three or four docs and was feeling hopeless, as each had told her that her despondency was "just stress" and "I can't find anything wrong with you." I could see what was happening—it was a familiar story—and for many, SSRIs were part of the solution, along with hormones. These were cases where low mood and lack of joy were the standout symptoms. Yet most women still fear the weight gain associated with antidepressants. So I always chose combinations of hormones and antidepressants that would have the least impact on appetite. I want women to find relief, and weight isn't just an emotional issue. If too much weight is going to hinder a woman's ability to exercise, that's also going to impact the quality of her Upgrade.

The key is individuality of dose and timing. Prozac, or "Vitamin P" as I like to call it, has the lowest impact on weight gain, and I found it to be the most flexible of the SSRIs. Average doses of Prozac for clinical depression are between 20 and 80 milligrams. But that's often way too high for women in the Transition. I liked to use the liquid form so I could help my patients microdose and find the best amount for them individually. I started many of my patients on doses from 2 to 5 milligrams. That's ten times less than the dose for clinical depression.

Whatever combination of HT and SSRI I prescribed, I started everyone on a tiny dose. We did test-drives of several formulas, starting small and increasing or decreasing slowly. We charted the dose and the timing, and patients recorded their feelings throughout the day, bringing those journals and charts to every visit. We even changed the time of the dose depending on those feelings. I wanted the women to have the best chance of the antidepressant cooperating with the body's natural rhythms and hormones. Those rhythms are in constant flux. Catching the right wave is crucial, and it takes time to figure out what works for you. I usually tell women it will take up to six months to get it right.

In the meantime, a new understanding of the neurochemical influence on mood is just beginning to emerge. For decades, the focus has been on SSRIs, drugs like Prozac that make serotonin more available. The thinking was that serotonin was what was needed to shift mood. New scientific techniques have allowed researchers to see that serotonin and dopamine are the two key players in mood, decision making, the reward system, depression, movement disorders, and thought disorders. It has thrown the field of treating mood and melancholy wide open. With the research being done into new compounds and approaches, I'm guessing we are going to see more effective treatments in the years to come.

Whether you opt for medical help or not, if you can calm the amygdala's and hypothalamus's alarm that pushes CRH, kicking off the body's threat-response system, it can help right the brain's ship. If we can find ways to increase the feelings of safety, nurturing, joy, it goes a long way to decreasing levels of cortisol and adrenaline. And tools for handling run-away negative rumination may save us from going down the road of intractable melancholy.

Think about Sarah's doctor and the recommendation to rest, be peaceful, and get some sleep. If she's feeling crappy because Insula 18.0 is torturing her over the fact that she can't run anymore, then she is being activated by threat, not safety. "I felt like a failure," Sarah said, "because I couldn't rest, and it seemed like I woke up progressively sadder every day. And then I tried to meditate with a friend. My mind wouldn't sit still. All I could think about was that this tiredness and bleeding would never end and that I would never get my life back. I felt like a complete failure."

Our female biology predisposes us to rumination because our stress system takes longer to downregulate; and Sarah got stuck in her sadness and self-flagellation. Remember, the brain has Velcro for negativity and Teflon for positivity. Any potential danger is perceived to be larger, and anything positive is dwarfed by it. If I wake up with a sequence of negative thoughts and scenes running through my head, they can take on a life of their own if I don't take action to put the brakes on rumination. It can ruin my morning, my day, even my mental health.

For me sometimes life events are so big that it's hard to focus, hard to settle down. So I make sure I find ways to get some distance from what's bothering me by taking a walk, exercising, or calling a friend to keep from crashing and burning on the altar of negativity. Deliberate breathing can also activate the cerebellum and trick the vagus nerve into signaling the parts of the nervous system that help us calm down. You can try alternate-nostril breathing or the box breathing that everybody is talking about. (See appendix, page 258.)

Tiny Muscles and Essential First Thoughts (EFTs)

When it comes to making change, I like to start small.

I have a new plan in the morning. I wake up, I wiggle my toes, and I smile, even if I don't feel like it, especially on the days I feel rotten, the hamster wheel of negative thoughts or worry already spinning off its axis by the time I open my eyes. Sometimes a scene from the past is there full blown on the viewing screen. If I stay there too long, then I will be sucked down the gravitational vortex of rumination about things that I can't change. Now I deploy my antinegativity missiles, like EFTs (essential first thoughts), better known as tools for coping. After that initial big, genuine smile, in which I make sure to engage my eyes, I imagine whatever force for goodness may be supporting our existence saying to me, "Good morning, Louann. I love you. I will be working for you today, and I won't be needing your help. Have a nice day. God." Emotionally, this helps me adjust expectations around what I am capable of controlling just for one day. Feeling cared for helps me make room for more kindness toward others. And much of that mood shift has to do with the neurobiological intervention of muscle movement.

It seems trivial to say that one way to improve your day is to wiggle your toes and smile first thing when you wake up, but each aspect of this new wake-up routine kicks off a positive neurological feedback loop that potentially reduces stress and inflammation. Anything that reduces inflammation helps the brain: Lower inflammation means preservation of cognition. The healthy effects get amplified as the seeds of friendliness impact relationships, which in turn helps me maintain the social connections that provide essential nutrition to my brain. It begins with the intentional firing of teeny tiny muscles like the levator anguli oris and zygomaticus, which raise the corners of the mouth, and the orbicularis oculi, which crinkle the eyes, the real signal to the brain and to others that the smile is not false but a genuine expression of warmth and friendship.

The theory that facial muscles can cause a shift in mood has been around since Darwin first wrote about it in 1872. Psychological studies over the course of the past fifty years continue to support the idea, and scientists have been trying to find the neurological trigger for just as long. Theories abound as to which facial nerves send the signal to the brain to begin its chemical cascade: facial muscle movement, nerves in facial skin, contraction or expansion of veins and arteries changing airflow in the nasal passages so that the brain detects a temperature change. Getting proof of how each mechanism works is still extremely hard, but based on what we know about the nervous system, it's impossible that there is no neurophysiological feedback loop operating here. Smiling, and making sure you involve the eyes, can elevate mood for a moment; even this can be enough of a window to feel a temporary release from difficult emotional states like uncertainty, melancholy, or even rage. Once that happens, we have opportunities to deploy more coping mechanisms, like balancing on one foot, which started a trajectory toward exercise and out of sadness for Rhonda.

Wiggling your toes activates the sciatic, the longest nerve in your body, sending a signal from the big toe to the sacrum and lumbar spine that gets the brain ready to wake up the legs and to move. The mound of the big toe is a powerful source of balance and stability as we stand and walk. It's the power behind every step, whether running or walking. It's the first place we bring our attention in any standing yoga posture to stabilize the pose and engage the legs. And wiggling your toes may activate circuits of fun, if you have memories of people playing with your toes and tickling your feet as a child. There are keys to cognition in moving our feet.

Flora's standard answer to "How are you?" was "Still kicking!" She meant that literally. Always a dancer, at age ninety-eight, she was in great shape. In her mideighties she started an elders tap-dancing troupe that visited senior-living communities to inspire others with their moves. "Dr. B.," she told me when I asked her how she kept up with all her activities, "as long as you keep moving, the buzzards won't get you." She was right, especially when it comes to supporting mental clarity. The neuromuscular feedback loops of movement are key to keeping the buzzards of declining cognition away.

Flora's "moving" and "kicking" are a key factor in her mental sharpness. A study of 120 older adults in Pittsburgh showed that consistent exercise, both aerobic and strength-training, changes the brain's anatomy by creating new cells and increasing the size of the hippocampus and the prefrontal cortex. That's a direct impact on the brain organs for memory, clearheaded thinking, and decision making. They are also the two brain areas most vulnerable to decline and aging.

Step ball change. Cross, cross. Skip and slide, jump and clap. Pump your arms, punch and curl, spin around. Balance and coordination challenge the cerebellum, which keeps signaling balance in emotion and judgment and the unleashing of creativity. Conquering a complex pattern stimulates the reward circuits, refreshing the cognitive centers in the brain. The intensity variation of starting and stopping also plays the adrenals to exhilaration, releasing just the right amount of the stress hormones to set off a cascade of neurochemical rewards, giving us that feeling that we can conquer the world. Intervals, even gentle ones, are key.

Before the Transition, going for a long run might have been one way of goosing endorphins to lift mood and brighten the mind. "I know I missed the high," said Sarah, lamenting that between exhaustion and arthritic hips, five-mile runs weren't an option anymore. "But my trainer gave me a twenty-minute interval program that was magical. [This can be modified to involve only the arms if you're having trouble walking.] There is a two-minute warm-up walk and then a sequence of four one-minute intervals: a fast walk, a slow jog, a faster jog or slow run, and a run at a pace I can handle. Repeat that four-minute cycle four times, ending with a two-minute walking cooldown. It seemed like nothing when she first described it, but I couldn't believe how quickly I was sweating! By the time I got to the middle of the second cycle of four minutes, I was feeling the kind of brain high that used to kick in around my second or third mile."

Here is what's happening to Sarah's brain. The adrenals pump a little cortisol, adrenaline, and norepinephrine, waking up just a little bit of vigilance as she completes the one-minute intervals. As soon as levels get just to the edge of stress, the adrenals are given a break; they calm down and stand down from kicking into high alert for fight or flight. The highs and lows of the cortisol waves mean that Sarah's brain doesn't get flooded with stress and inflammation. On the contrary, it's just enough to ask for the dopamine and endorphin neurochemical release that makes exercise so joyful—a runner's high without the exhausting run. You can apply intervals like this to any aerobic exercise: cycling, walking outside, rowing, arm cycles (especially important for anyone wheelchair bound), swimming. Dance has intervals in its DNA.

I knew that Sarah had had a bout with pneumonia that left her in bed for six weeks, so I asked her what she did to get back to exercise. "Did you use the same routine?"

"In a way I did," she said. "But I modified it with help. When I was younger, I would have tried to come back with the same intensity on day one, and probably would have gotten away with it. But since the Transition I have learned to start more slowly. So instead of basing the intervals on pace, we used incline. I kept the walking pace slow, used a flat incline for the warm-up and cooldown, and steadily increased the incline through the four minutes, starting over each time at the lower level. It took a month to get a little energy back, and two months before I was ready to jog a little. Now I'm switching it up even more. I'm focusing on things like cardio dance and adding barre classes with light weights and Pilates. Combining them, I find I burn more calories and I'm more exhilarated by exercise instead of being drained."

After just one exercise session, your brain responds by putting out more neurotransmitters like endorphin, dopamine, noradrenaline, and serotonin, all of which raise your mood as soon as you towel off, and this becomes protective against persistent melancholy. A single workout is capable of amping up our ability to focus for at least two hours afterward and improves reaction time—it's a great weapon against reflexes slowing with age. And even if you haven't been very physically active before, exercise will bring benefits at any age. A study of 8,206 women from the Women's Health Initiative showed that women who started working out at ages seventy to seventy-nine benefited after just twelve weeks.

Movement reminds the cerebellum that it has to keep the automatic functions strong; otherwise it will begin to close the shop. When movement is limited, the cerebellum isn't pinged as much to stimulate other functions, such as emotion regulation and problem-solving. The nervous system's activation and motivation for basic survival of the body declines. The heart and lungs and cardiovascular system don't get the signal that they need to function optimally in order to support life. Muscles aren't stressed in a way that builds them; the brain, in turn, gets a weaker signal to maintain heart, lungs, and circulation to support basic nervous-system needs for survival. It doesn't take long for the downward spiral to begin.

Without movement, muscles begin to waste. Called sarcopenia, this wasting can become the enemy of balance, and it's often an indicator that severe cognitive decline is not far behind. Muscle loss, like bone loss, actually starts soon after age thirty but can become a rapid, progressive, debilitating condition after age sixty unless muscle-strengthening exercises are done. Within twenty-four hours of being bedridden, muscle fibers start to lose strength. If you're in bed for several weeks, you lose muscle strength at a rate of about 12 percent a week. After three to five weeks of bed rest, almost half of the normal strength of a muscle is gone. I remember that feeling after my hip replacement. It comes back fast, but you have to take small steps; if you jump back in too fast, injury and pain put you back to square one.

A study in Sweden found that in people aged sixty to eighty, the more fit someone was, as measured by a session on a stationary bike, the more words they were able to mentally access. In animal trials, we're finding that exercise significantly increases the number of new neurons being made in a few critical parts of the brain, meaning: neurogenesis! It is possible to make new neurons at any age, and exercise helps bulk up the parts of the brain that can protect us from memory loss and cognitive decline. The female brain is begging us to work out in the Upgrade. It's time to answer the call.

If you've been sitting too much, the core muscles of the body begin to atrophy, and the glutes—our butt muscles, which power forward motion— get a kind of amnesia. Crucial to the movement behind getting up out of a chair, they forget to do their job, putting our balance and the cerebellum at risk. If you've been putting off a knee or hip replacement, it's time to get it done for the sake of your brain. If you've been too sedentary, like sitting in a chair for hours at the computer like me, squeeze your butt and change your brain. Twenty chair squats a day, and then a hundred butt squeezes (squeeze for three counts, relax for three counts). Break them into batches of twenty-five if you have to. I do mine while brushing my teeth. You can do them sitting, standing, or lying down. But doing them will fuel your centers of balance and judgment.

So move those toes, stand up, and when you get to the bathroom, stop at the mirror. Smile at yourself. Get the muscles around your eyes into the act. Using the mirror engages the visual cortex, the largest part of the brain, and starts a neurological feedback loop that elicits joy. It only takes ten to fifteen seconds of your own eyes twinkling back at you to make an impact, so forget about the crow's-feet. In fact, wrinkle them as much as possible. When, during the day, the brain serves up random uncomfortable thoughts that have nothing to do with reality, reigniting the memory of the feeling from the morning is usually enough to keep them from ruining your day.

Your body knows that movement will signal your brain, *I am alive and well,* and that well-being follows it. It craves movement snacks. They can be five or ten minutes if you're too busy to do a sustained workout or don't have access. Get up and walk around the house during commercials if you're watching TV. Park a good distance from where you need to go, if you can. Get off public transportation a stop early, or walk to the next one to pick it up. Do ten chair squats whenever you can. Some of us need help remembering to take a movement snack, especially if we are stuck inside or at a desk. Get a reminder app, or if you have a smart watch, turn on the reminders to stand and move, and try to be compliant. Your brain will reward you with sharpness, alertness, and protection of cognition that will last longer. If you want to boost your sharpness, the effects of a moderate burst of exercise are strongest for the first two hours afterward. If you are not able to take HT, we now know that movement provides a massive boost to brain health. And if you are on HT, studies are indicating that fitness not only boosts the effects of estrogen on the brain but offsets risks associated with HT as well.

If you haven't moved in a while, or if you're recovering from surgery or an illness, microdose at the beginning. Walk around your dining room table. Then move it up to hallways, until you have the stamina to walk around the block. Do it every single day. After you build strength, ramp up your distance slowly, and your energy will rise exponentially. If you aren't mobile enough to walk, exercise your arms. Raise them up and move them for a few minutes. Build up to five, then ten. Turn on a symphony and conduct it. Feel the joy of play again. Your body and brain are begging you for it!

The Return of Purpose

Chapter 12

Around the dining room table overlooking Manhattan's East River sat several women, among them two former media executives, a (current) venture capitalist, a former White House counsel, a former curator at one of the world's most important art museums, and a designer who had done iconic work that made her famous. Among them ages ranged between near fifty and early seventies. The collective body blows around the table included loss of children, spouses, careers, money, social status, health, looks, and community support. Each woman would tell you she had been torn down to the bone, pride stripped, life shattered. Everything each once held dear had been released, including old strategies—drinking, travel, shopping, excessive exercise, and obsessive self-improvement—to acquire peace. Everything that they had once thought essential to survival and success no longer seemed important.

Though their lives and origins looked very different—hailing from European upper-class to Hollywood, from mid-Atlantic working class to middle-class Manhattan native—all of them agreed on one point. The blows life had delivered provided the best opportunity to step into who they really are. "I wouldn't trade most of these experiences for anything in the world," said Jean, who had lost her husband. "Hardship has made me who I am. Not a drop of it was easy or fun, and if you'd have told me any of this at the time, I probably would have decked you."

"Yes, there's nothing more infuriating than someone coming at you with spiritual pablum like 'You'll see this will be a blessing,'" Marian interjected. "Especially when you're midtrauma. People can be really unskillful, even if what they are saying might turn out to be true. It takes time to heal, time for the trauma of it all to unwind."

Nancy, now in her late sixties, was a legendary beauty. She was interviewed by a national newspaper along with two actresses who were complaining about losing their looks. But she didn't see aging as a drawback; in fact she was thrilled. "For the first time in my life, I can get a man to listen to and accept my ideas and advice," she said. No longer pulling male attention meant Nancy could begin to get things done even with men in the room.

As for the others, many found new careers, found new communities, and started their own businesses. They allowed tough times to bring out their best, relishing their ability to meet a struggle, even when it was hard. They found purpose again, and not a bit of it was driven by anyone or anything outside their own internal engine. In no longer having anything to lose, they found in the Full Upgrade the freedom to be and do what was most authentically aligned with who they are.

The attention we paid over our lifetimes—no matter our level of achievement in the world—to hair, makeup, clothes, was part of nature's brainwashing that these rituals were what would attract a mate and get our genes reproduced. All that primping is part of nature's strategy around propagation of the species.

The wiring of fertility's survival imperative keeps us restless, always seeking satisfaction and approval from the outside. It locks us in an excruciating tension—*It worked! He's checking me out!* and *He only likes me for my breasts.* The internal scream *This isn't all of me!* is nearly impossible to stifle. It was certainly hard for me. Even though intellectually we may know appearance isn't everything, the feeling that if we are not attractive we will die is real: Nature makes sure you will believe a delusion if it means you'll find someone to reproduce with. That includes picking the wrong person. So right now you can forgive yourself many of the errors in judgment during the fertility years. We've all made mistakes. The misperceptions about relationships, the misreadings of character, the lopsided priorities, were designed to a degree by natural selection. Getting stuck in those old stories can be an off-ramp into a downgrade.

By the time you've reached the Transition, the selfish gene-survival imperative to reproduce itself is over. In the Upgrade, that game is over. And with it comes a new beginning, with new rules and a survival imperative that drives a new sense of purpose. It's different for everyone.

"I was shocked by how my thinking changed," said seventy-year-old Alina. "I've done corporate interiors most of my life, but everything changed when I had grandchildren. It's like my heart exploded and my sense of protectiveness extended to all children. It was completely spontaneous. I couldn't look at another child without thinking, *This is my grandchild, too.* And right after that came the thought *Shit, we have wrecked the planet! How will they survive? I need to do something to protect the grandchildren now!*"

Alina was still running her firm but started spending much more time engaged with environmental and political activism. "I am a fierce recycler, and my local and state representatives are sick of hearing from me about enforcing the laws. But I don't care. This is too important."

Alina had had insomnia during the Transition, so I wondered how she was faring these days. "How are you sleeping with all this on your plate?" I asked.

"Actually, I'm happier, more energetic, and more focused than I've felt in years," she said. "Staying engaged with something that matters so much has given my life new meaning."

Alina's engaged, purpose-driven mindset was also activating protective circuitry in the brain that blocks depression. Whether or not those circuits are activated can be shaped by the decision made when faced with the fork in the Transition road that some women face: heed the siren call to exit into the comfortable Transition, or build your Upgrade.

Life Extension

Jane, at fifty-four, realized she was only ever going to have one grandchild. It was a tremendous sadness at first because she loves children. Instead of grieving, she went back to school for a degree in social work and, finding new purpose, became an infant mental health specialist and a play therapist. "It meant I could go into preschools and play with kids all day long," she said, beaming. "Meanwhile, I was helping to keep at-risk kids from becoming at-risk teens and at-risk adults. If you intervene early with cognitive, behavioral, and emotional issues, you can change the course of a person's life."

The stimulation of the joy circuits through regular play was magical fuel. Over time, she built a foundation that focused on helping families, toddlers, and preschool teachers create the best learning environment possible in underserved neighborhoods. At seventy-five she's handed the reins to a younger director, but she is still engaged with educating educators and adults in foster-grandparenting programs. "I just can't seem to get myself to stop. I love it."

It's long been known that finding purpose and having a direction for your life lowers mortality risk beyond other factors that impact longevity, like a healthy diet and lifestyle. With diet and lifestyle, the sooner you begin, the greater the impact on your protection from disease. Researchers in Canada assumed the same would be true for purpose and embarked on a study to confirm their assumption. They were sure that the earlier you discover purpose, the bigger the impact on your health. But the biggest surprise in the fourteen-year follow-up period was that finding your purpose had the same benefits to longevity regardless of the age of discovery. Looking at six thousand participants, it was clear: Age didn't matter when it comes to the return of purpose, and purpose might even be more health protective in older adults than it is in younger ones. It's never too late to start asking questions around what you feel you were meant to do. In the Upgrade you'll finally have the bandwidth to do it, even though you might have trouble remembering things.

Engaging in purpose to fuel the Upgrade is a choice that's not always so clear. In 2016, when I handed over my role at the UCSF Women's Mood and Hormone Clinic, a part of me felt a huge relief. For the first time in decades, the weight of taking care of students and patients, training new staff, and raising money for my program and the institution was off my shoulders. I felt like I could breathe. And I did. As I stared out over San Francisco Bay, I started taking photos. Liking what I saw, I got interested in learning real technique and using a real camera. So I took classes and got a lot of validation. I even had a couple of exhibits. I went into a state of joy for several years, getting into a creative flow, learning a new skill set, and hanging out with artists instead of doctors. I learned oil painting and textile design, things I loved when I was young. It felt like I was picking up a dropped stitch in the knitting of my life. But I didn't realize that the comfortable Transition was a bit of a dead end.

I got to a point where I realized that the only way forward with photography would be to study a lot of technical stuff in Photoshop, and that just wasn't what I wanted to do with my life. I was missing the outward orientation of my profession, the interactional interdependence and intimate engagement of caring for patients. I had felt euphoric doing art, but—boom!—just like that I was depressed and alone, bereft of the colleagues, life, and career I had spent decades building. Just like wrinkles and watermelon boobs, I had always thought, *This is not going to happen to me,* and then—surprise!—isolation and uselessness busted down the door. Like the transitional men I had dated between marriages, even though the relationships felt real and all-consuming at first, I had to recognize that art was a phase, the comfortable Transition. There were more meaningful things I was meant to take care of, like helping other women access the Upgrade.

I like to think in pie charts. When I think about the brain bandwidth that the survival imperative—*stay healthy and attractive in order to mate and reproduce*—took up in the fertility era, it was almost the entire pie. Neurohormones were screaming at us to put most of our attention on everything that supports fertility—relationships, looks, fitness. But if I look at the pie chart of the survival imperative for the Upgrade, it's blue sky for new priorities. It's blue sky for purpose, for turning the arrow of concern outward. This is a major ingredient for joy in the brain.

If my survival-imperative pie chart is taken up with a narrow, fearful version of the question, like a constant refrain of *What's going to happen to me?*, then I might be setting myself up for depression. Yes, I have to be practical about taking care of myself, but if my time is spent worrying about what I'm losing or how I'm going to struggle to hang on to what's past, then I may be activating the neurocircuitry for depression. When the arrows of concern only point inward toward ourselves, we can hit bottom pretty fast. In extreme cases, too much self-concern can activate debilitating states that can keep us from functioning, like profound melancholy and even obsessive-compulsive disorder. But flip the arrow outward, make the survival-imperative pie chart focus on engaging with things that matter to others, and we become connected and energetic. Purpose reemerges.

This opposite of self-cherishing, focusing on others, is for me as good as it gets, and the neurochemicals and circuitry that get turned on explain why that is. When advanced meditators were studied in fMRIs, they were asked to cultivate compassion, the empathetic mental state of wanting to be of help to others. During their meditations, the minute this compassion arose from their hearts, the joy circuits in the brain's region of higher thinking exploded. This isn't the same thing as being a martyr or a doormat. Those feelings don't bring joy in the brain. They bring frustration and probably some negative self-talk. You can't obliterate yourself and be helpful at the same time. You have to bring your whole calm, clearheaded being to the table. You have to have no agenda other than being helpful.

Finding the right fit, the best way forward in returning to purpose after leaving a work environment, can be incredibly challenging, not only to the tent of "Me" but in terms of options presented by the culture.

When men leave big positions, they are generally offered paid board seats and consulting gigs that aren't available to women. "You get asked to volunteer," said Alina. "You get asked to give a lot of free advice. But a paying gig? I know a lot of men who got them, but even my most powerful female friends have struggled with the fact that they are expected to be corporate caretakers and work for free."

It doesn't matter where you worked, what your career was, or if you worked. You will be asked to volunteer, while men of a similar age will be paid. There are plenty of resources for connecting older people to volunteer opportunities, but what about the woman with no means? A woman whose care for elderly parents drained her resources after her husband left her and then she lost her job? "I was aged out of my job at the bank a year ago," said Carole. "All I wanted was another job, but I was chased by every major advocacy organization to sit on their boards for free. The ladies who lunch," she continued, "expected me to contribute my knowledge to their causes for free, to do all their finances for free, but I was a lady who still needed to make money to pay for that lunch. The feeling of isolation during that time was profound."

The isolation of female professionals in the Upgrade is real. During our careers, colleagues can feel closer than blood relatives, but many find that when we are downsized or retire, that social world evaporates. Men have experienced this, but this emotional gut punch is new in history for women; it's a new developmental stage that, if left unaddressed, can keep us stuck in Transition-mind or Early Upgrade.

The minute you're out of the loop, all the old junior high school circuits of feeling left out by the popular kids are reactivated. No matter how high your social status, no matter how elevated your success, it happens. "Even in my activism," said Alina, "if I discover I've been left out of a meeting, it puts me right back to the twelve-year-old girl who wasn't invited to the cool kids' party."

During her Transition and Upgrade, remember that Sherry surprised herself by taking a bunch of exercise classes to meet new people after moving from the East Coast to Arizona to be with her son David and his family. But she also found new purpose. "One of the ways I pulled myself out of sadness after moving to Arizona to be with David and the grandkids was to become a consultant to café and restaurant owners," she recalled. "I charged a small fee for helping them create structure and organization around the business side. I was mostly working from home at the time. Many of my meetings were by video chat. When I realized I was going to classes because I missed having colleagues, I found an office to rent in a fantastic co-working space for entrepreneurs who had been running a business for three or more years. Most of the tenants were women and minority business owners, and that was magic. Through new connections and hallway conversations, I rediscovered what I loved about my work and started my first growth spurt after having left the East Coast. That growth was driven by my hiring subcontractors, women out there struggling on their own who needed to reignite their confidence, their skills, and even their careers. Seeing how many women I was starting to help, well, that made me pop out of bed every day."

Clearing the Obstacle of Worry

The pre-Upgrade female brain is wired to see danger everywhere, to be on high alert to protect the helpless around her. High waves of estrogen and the stress hormone cortisol keep this instinct front and center, inhibiting access to questions that seem less like life-and-death, and more like *What should I do with my life after the Transition?* Not only is this not an issue for the male brain, but testosterone makes men much more tolerant of risk. The higher the testosterone, the less they perceive risk. If you've partnered with a man, or been in a car with a couple that's been together for a long time, you have heard the difference of perception of risk manifest in an old, familiar argument. "For god's sake, slow down! You're going to kill us all! The kids are in the car!" "Honey, what are you talking about? I'm driving just fine. When's the last time I had an accident? Never. That's right. Now stop criticizing me."

The difference in the perception of risk is estrogen keeping the female brain hypervigilant to danger in its drive to protect the vulnerable ones. When hormonal waves calm and estrogen lowers, it dials down that constant alertness.

With the quieting of the hormonal siren call to worry, there is more silence in which to hear our own voice. There is more room in our mind for the return of purpose. The answers to who we are and how we want to live become clearer.

It will seem unfamiliar at first, the urge to explore the world alone, to start a business—*What am I doing at my age?*—to climb mountains and fly solo. But once you start taking new adventures, you become addicted. "Grandma, can I come with you to Japan?" While at times you may say yes, at other times you might feel, *Are you kidding? My worst nightmare! I just want to do this by myself.* You say, "Oh, honey, not this time. You would be bored with this old lady. Maybe the next trip."

Being on purpose brings all the parts of yourself into focus. Work becomes mission driven; curiosity takes center stage in decision making; a new ease, even in difficult moments, takes over. It doesn't mean that the worry circuits never turn on again—I have certainly struggled with that in regard to my son, and that may never change. But there is enough release to start exploring new ways to engage with proactively undoing a lifetime of brainwashing about who we are and what we can contribute.

Keeping Purpose on Track

When I was a child, things pretty much went my way. Of course I had my traumas, but I was the smartest kid in class and successful at most things I tried. However, then I got my period and reality changed. What struck me to my core was the deep unfairness of my own biology, that I was going to have this for what seemed like the rest of my life and boys would never have to experience it. When my biology announced itself, I was unprepared for it, even though I was educated about it. I didn't know how dramatically cramps and moodiness would alter my world for days each month. I had a similar experience during pregnancy, when morning sickness came with a nausea so powerful it shut out the rest of existence. And then the neurochemicals of motherhood rewired my brain for overprotectiveness and a deep dread of relationship rupture with my child and my spouse.

Evolutionary biologist Richard Dawkins wrote a seminal book in the

1970s called *The Selfish Gene*. In it he argues that the only thing Mother Nature cares about is getting sperm into the next generation, ergo that's all men care about. The book that needs to be written about women's biology is *The Unselfish Gene*. Think about it. Since a mother and baby don't have matching DNA, the female immune system has to be suppressed so that the baby doesn't die. The Upgrade is the first time in a woman's life she doesn't have to biologically or psychologically suppress something so that another may survive. But the social expectation that she will continue to do this, and to suppress her own purpose, remains. Thus the burden of caretaking, which she expects of herself as well. It falls on women as inevitably as puberty.

"I remember being so overwhelmed," said Mariana, fifty-two. "My mother-in-law had a stroke and had been taken to rehab. I was the primary breadwinner; my husband's accounting practice had hit the rocks while my career was soaring. But the nurses and social workers wouldn't talk to him or his brother. They waited for me to visit and they asked me, not them, 'So what's the plan for how you will take care of her after she is discharged?' I had no idea what to do. And I had no idea that my now-ex-husband would actually be useless. So was his brother. I was earning all the money, and I became responsible for things like picking up her laundry from rehab, which was an hour away, taking it home, washing it, and bringing it back. I ended up being in charge of managing caretakers when she moved in with us. It was another full-time job. I was so busy that I had to turn down a bunch of opportunities for career growth. I ended up blowing a promotion."

I hear this all the time. Chantal, fifty, a former news anchor, roared in frustration when her brother refused to help her care for their mother when she was diagnosed with Alzheimer's. Chantal's mother lived with her until it became unmanageable. She sobbed the day she signed an agreement with a facility. It was a combination of despair over feeling she hadn't done enough and the loneliness of the process. Chantal had been building her own media business while cleaning up after her mother's incontinence, responding to 3:00 A.M. demands for dinner, and putting her child through college. All of her friends saw that she was squeezing out her last ounce of love, strength, and care. It was outrageous to her friends to think she was awash in guilt and remorse over failing her mother, yet those feelings were so real and so solid. That's an indication of a mommy-brain-circuit reality hijack, one that brings shame and social isolation with it. The gift of hearing the hard truth from a friend—that there was nothing more anyone else could have done and that her brother was a class-A jerk—is part of what got her back out into the world.

For some women, caretaking is purpose, it's a career, it's life; that's not what I'm talking about here. I'm talking about how much of it women get saddled with without choosing it consciously. Most of us talk about being cared for at home in our final days, but if there isn't a woman around to make sure it happens, who will do it? If you are a woman with dementia who was abandoned by her partner and you have only brothers, who will care for you? How will it be paid for? Just as 78 percent of childcare is done by women—even if they have full-time jobs—the same thing has to be true of the other end of life. They don't keep statistics on it yet, and that is an indication of just how pervasive this unspoken expectation is.

It's a blinding reflex for some of us. My patient Natalie, sixty-three, can have a chockablock-full calendar, but if there is a caretaking need, it's as though the clouds part and her schedule becomes clear blue sky. She's let herself take sole responsibility for her elderly parents, her mother-in-law, and her sister-in-law who had a stroke in her fifties. There are siblings and spouses, but she does it all. It's hard for her to resist what I call the helper circuits.

From the time we are teeny tiny, "Help Mommy with this, please" is a siren call to feel useful. Many in our lives count on those helper-brain circuits being activated when they mindlessly call out, "Where's the . . ." or "How do I . . . ," to suck us into helping them with minutiae that pull us off task and out of our own zone of purpose, as though we were the family's Google, on call and available 24-7.

Before getting married, Natalie had a career with an international management consulting firm, one she didn't want to give up, but felt she had to in order to help her husband grow his burgeoning and extremely successful fitness franchise. She designed events for big meetings and top franchisees while raising the kids and caring for the older generation. "I see my daughter with her kids, a career, and a partner who fully participates in the caretaking, and I think about what I gave up that she didn't have to," Natalie tells me. "It's hard. Motherfucker, it's what I wanted. I take those feelings out, look at them, and then stuff them back inside, because really, what else can I do?" The fear that she'll be criticized if she doesn't do it all is overwhelming. But there is real evidence that caretaking stress not only is an obstacle to the return of purpose but may shorten a woman's life.

Part of the way we keep living is that cells replicate. At the end of the strands of DNA that make up chromosomes are telomeres, a kind of protective cap that keeps the ends of chromosomes from fraying and making them sticky. The common image used is the plastic on the end of a shoelace. Intact telomeres are essential to healthy genetic material. Science now has a way to measure telomeres; the longer they are, the lower the impact of aging on all cells, including brain and nervous system cells. A 2014 study done on unpaid female family caregivers in Wisconsin showed significant shortening of telomeres. Conclusion: Caretaker stress accelerates aging.

From the outside, Natalie looks like one of the most badass women you'll ever meet. But scratch the surface and you find she is exhausted and often bedridden from caregiving fatigue. It doesn't come without reward. There is gratification in being in the space of compassion, because of the positive feedback women get socially and culturally for overly developed empathy and guilt circuits. We get to be the rescuer, everyone approves, we get a dopamine reward for success, and so we become chronic, daily rescuers. Purpose gets buried once again, unless caretaking is the chosen path for it.

The expectations of the culture will fall on you as inevitably as your biology. I had no choice about my period, but there is a choice about caretaking. If we know to question it before it happens, to recruit others and make a plan ahead of time, we have a chance to live the second half the way we envision it, not hijacked by and drowning in biological and sociological guilt. Of course, in the thick of it you will have to change some of your plans. It's inevitable that your care for an ill partner or close family member will change the dynamics. But it's good to have a plan and some backup help, so that caretaking can become episodic rather than chronic.

Awakening Purpose by Speaking Up

In my childhood, there was no fiercer truth teller than my grandmother. She'd spill the family secrets at Thanksgiving and in front of everyone ask a cousin why he snuck that cookie when he'd been told not to take one before dinner—*yes, of course she saw him*. Everyone attributed her lack of inhibition to eccentricity or a possibly failing mind. But this wasn't the case for my grandmother. It was simply the lifting of the hormonal shroud of accommodation, allowing her to find a new comfort in her own skin.

As young girls, say four to six years old, chances are we were scolded more than once for using our outdoor voice to tell an older relative they had bad breath, or they were fat, or they had a mole that looked gross. We spoke out not only because we weren't yet properly socialized; we spoke out because the brain circuits for judgment and especially conflict avoidance hadn't yet come online. We don't yet know how or why it happens, but during puberty the female brain changes dramatically. The amygdala, a center for fear and anger response, develops more in puberty and is triggered easily by estrogen and testosterone. Since men have more testosterone, their anger and physical aggression are triggered more readily together. But for women, with higher estrogen and much less testosterone, the signals to leap into battle are less direct. When the fertility cycle begins in earnest, the effect is that an outspoken little girl suddenly becomes a confused, frustrated, and sad preteen, especially when you ask her to explain what's wrong.

Nature selected for this characteristic: In the wild, a lower aggression flash point probably meant better chances of survival for the smaller gender. Starting fistfights with much larger primitive males probably wasn't a great bet for success, so evolution wired a lock on the dam of female aggression. As estrogen lowers in the Upgrade, this lock on aggression can open. The part of the brain that used to hijack anger and strangle our voice is now neurologically released. Given the female acuity with language, we are more likely to throw words instead of fists. No more mulling over what to do or say. A gusher of well-timed zingers can blow, and so Grandma starts telling you the truth. She reads situations and acts.

In trying to categorize the Upgrade's new freedom, I often hear women talking about recovering the girl we left behind, her attitudes, and her behaviors. But that implies nothing has happened since you were eight. A lifetime of hormonal waves has changed your brain circuits. A lifetime of experience has brought wisdom. There may be dreams and hopes and wishes that ache to be pulled forward, but it doesn't mean you are going back. It means that you are finally able to incorporate that girl into who you are now, instead of leaving her abandoned by the side of the road. It can mean integrating her drive to fuel the return of purpose.

The voice in our head that used to censor us, always telling us to be quiet so that we didn't offend or upset anyone, becomes less loud in the Upgrade. We are less pulled by our peripheral vigilance over the needs of others, and we can discover a power pack we didn't know we had. All that power is difficult to control at first, so don't be surprised by sudden explosions. It can be like driving on a racetrack with a Maserati after decades of struggling to get a bald-tired VW Beetle up an icy hill. This force is necessary. If a child is walking into traffic, there is nothing gentle about the bellowed warning or the force needed to push that child out of harm's way. If we need to carve out the space for the return of purpose, to be our authentic selves, it's essential. It's powerful. It's fiercely female.

"No" Is a Complete Sentence

"I'm sorry," said Lisa, sixty-five, after speaking her mind. I was staying in her large home, and I was one of three houseguests. As the chef/owner of a restaurant, she was doing all the cooking for us. She had asked that, after four days of nonstop meal preparation, we figure out dinner on our own. She was tired, and we all had cars and the means to go out. Making that request felt like anger to her, but to the rest of us, not only did it sound reasonable, but we felt a little guilty that we hadn't offered to bring in food for everyone sooner.

Lisa and I sat at the kitchen table overlooking the woods behind her house. Over a cup of tea, I asked her about that apology for setting what I perceived to be a healthy boundary. "It felt super aggressive," she said. "I felt angry. It just burst out of me, and I thought I hurt everyone's feelings."

I could understand where she was coming from, but none of us experienced her as being angry. It was clear she was overloaded, and I wondered why she had agreed to cook meals for so many people for so many days. Looking down at her cup of tea, she said, "It just never occurred to me that I could say no."

One of the most important lessons I've learned in the Upgrade, specifically in keeping purpose on track, is that "No" is a complete sentence. But it's one we might not have spoken with confidence since we were toddlers.

"No" is for many children their first word. We don't have to learn this assertion of will; we are born knowing how to signal distress, whether verbally or physically, by squirming, using our arms and legs to escape something uncomfortable or threatening. From two years old on, we were taught to stuff our "no," opening the door to shattered boundaries and choices that might not be right for us. Is it any surprise that by the time we reach the Upgrade we almost don't know where to find it? Or that it bursts out when you least expect it, catches you by surprise? It can feel like you have no idea where it came from, like it was somewhere deep inside, stored in the nervous system's lockbox. When it emerges in the Upgrade, it comes through the tempered steel of age, not out of a childhood stubbornness. This is not a reversion. It's an integration, a reweaving of the part of ourselves our culture and biology told us to pack away.

In the fertility phase I felt compelled to say yes to everything, squeezing too much into the corset of each day. At some point "yes" breaks you and every promise you've made to yourself about how you want to live.

You didn't need to learn to say no as a toddler. But who taught you to say no as a woman? If you can't remember, that is a problem that we need to fix now, in this uncharted, post-Transition developmental stage. I had to relearn this lesson myself if I was going to be healthy enough to stick to my new plan of getting back to books and back to helping women. I was in horrible pain from a pinched nerve in my neck when I got on a plane to visit a friend in New Mexico. This pain wasn't new—it had been lingering for almost a month, and I was incapacitated by it. I sat through therapy sessions pinching my other side to distract myself from the pain so that I could be present to others. Knowing my friend was looking forward to the time together on a big birthday, I didn't want to disappoint her, so I said yes and made the trip when I should have simply stated, "This isn't good for me right now." I was trying to work on this book, and it turned out to be a massive disruption.

It was a wake-up call that with every request I have to remember to run these questions through my brain and body: *Is this good for me? Is this good for living on purpose?* We usually override that doubt about adding another responsibility with *I'm being selfish; I can handle extra pain; this is more important than my own pain.* But at a certain point, we will run through our reserves; muscling through now comes with serious consequences. Sincerely asking ourselves the question *Is this good for me?* can be scary, because sometimes a truthful answer will mean a fight or rupture if others aren't used to hearing "no." But in the Upgrade, we no longer put our health, well-being, and living on purpose second.

I had to coach myself to say no by watching women who do it well. I started by writing down phrases that got me more comfortable with not saying yes. Practicing got my brain and nervous system used to a new response. When I didn't feel comfortable saying no right off the bat, I responded by saying, "Let me sleep on that and I'll get back to you." It gave me time to gather the courage. And if I wasn't able to get that phrase out and immediately regretted agreeing to something I didn't want to do, then I would say something like "On second thought, I need to sleep on that" or "On second thought, let me check my calendar" (or talk with my family, etc.).

Setting boundaries that help us protect our purpose might be biologically harder for women to do. Everything about the wiring of the female brain is about connecting, and that includes our threat response. It's been more than twenty years since researchers at UCLA discovered that women respond differently from men to stress. We don't just get a burst of cortisol and adrenaline triggering the fight-or-flight response and firing up our muscles; the bonding hormone oxytocin is also part of the female stress response. When faced with threat, we will do everything we can to maintain relationships. This female stress response is called tend and befriend.

If you've ever gotten into a fight with a child, spouse, or close friend and found yourself compulsively insistent on talking things out until you felt okay with the relationship, it's likely oxytocin driving that urge to make peace immediately. It's the imprints from waves of fertility hormones and an echo of life on the savanna, when a ruptured relationship could mean death in exile. When the waves calm in the Upgrade and that intense drive to bond no longer overwhelms our brain, we can find some freedom for purpose if we can overcome decades of neurochemically driven habits.

The quieting of the tend-and-befriend neurohabit helps create respectful space in relationships. When we don't rush in to fix, resolve, and control, all parties have a chance to let their stress circuits calm and the decision-making process reignite. A side effect is that we honor the other person's process. Just ask your spouse and kids if that tend-and-befriend, we-need-to-talk thing feels invasive. They will tell you it does. It takes a kind of fierce confidence to let go and trust that with time and distance things will work themselves out.

There is a learning curve on pushback, and one of the things we discover is that when handled straightforwardly, it brings respect, not the dislike we fear. Think about those you know who stand their ground well: Aren't they women you respect? If you've thought of yourself as a pleaser your whole life, then this will be a struggle. But the liberation is amazing. Just think back over all the times you wished you'd said no, the times of feeling buried under the mountain of "yeses," the mountain of regrets over not saying no. It's time to push back on demands. It can change the way we live the second half of our lives.

Making Friends with Boredom: The Discovery of Purpose

Remember, hormones are molecules that drive behavior, so when estrogen and testosterone drop, that sense of persistent striving releases its grip as well. When the hormonal waves quieted for me in the Upgrade, everything felt odd. I had just left the clinic, and after a lifetime of constantly reacting and responding to my role, I couldn't shut that habit off. I had ideaphoria. Millions of ideas were popping up, and I chased each one like a squirrel collecting acorns. I would report each new one to my husband, Sam, along with the progress I'd made in pursuing it, and he would say, "Louann's going fast nowhere." It took me a while to realize that my brain and nervous system resisted adjusting to the lack of schedule and role. That new lack of stimulus registered as boredom. And boredom really frightened me at first.

The first step in the return of purpose is to learn that boredom won't kill you, though the shift will make you feel like something is wrong—remember, the brain and nervous system love the familiar. With boredom comes not death but stillness. Being able to sit with uncertainty about how my life would unfold became crucial to the unfolding of new purpose. Facing the essential boredom of figuring out what you will do with the second half will be necessary whether you've worked inside or outside the home.

There are secrets in boredom. All kinds of things can come up, old memories, old triggers, long-buried dreams, long-buried regrets. It's like opening that neglected storage closet that's full of everything you threw in there that you didn't want to deal with at the time. You don't have to organize and clean that closet all at once. You may only need to look once and do nothing. Or you may take it a little at a time. Bite off what you can chew. There is no need for heroics in the Upgrade.

To keep myself from spinning out over every new idea, a friend helped me to just celebrate that my brain could generate so many. It helped me to watch each idea arise and smile as it floated away. If it came back, I considered it again, but mostly they were just a product of my nervous system churning in response to the unfamiliar stillness.

The answer to the question of your purpose may not be immediately clear. So many of us didn't know that asking what we want at this stage would be an option. It may be belonging, love, friendship, quiet. It may be activism, a new career, a new role in the family. Don't be frightened if you don't know right away. The answers will come in silence.

New Focus

Chapter 13

My friend Diane, a successful internist at a large private health system, had come of age after the first wave of feminism. She entered adulthood with the expectation of having it all—a fulfilling career and family. But the details of exactly how to juggle everything had never been ironed out, and she had found herself *doing* it all, never thinking she could ask for help. Between raising her kids, managing the household, and her work as a doctor, she had little time left to focus on her marriage or cultivate close friendships. She hit the Transition feeling lost and alone, in a fog of anxiety and difficulty in concentrating at work.

But the Upgrade was a different story. She felt stronger and more focused than perhaps ever in her life. Her kids had launched their own lives, she started reconnecting with old friends, and she tabled her efforts to "fix" her marriage. *Who knows,* she thought, *maybe I'll decide to leave. Maybe things will change.* She could finally stop juggling.

She threw herself into her career with a vigor she hadn't felt since medical school. Every case fascinated her; every patient interaction felt new. She found herself drawing on her wealth of experience to support her views and decisions; she dropped the second-guessing of the Transition for the careful analysis of the Upgrade. For the first time, she saw the younger women around her not as a threat to her position but as a new generation to be mentored and sponsored. She found a new focus in her Upgraded circuitry.

Waves of fertility hormones can increase stress hormones. The more stress hormones we have, the more threatening things seem. It's easier, during the fertile phase and the Transition, to tip into overwhelm. And the part of the brain that controls attention shifting—i.e., multitasking— gets overloaded and attention to detail begins to erode. The feeling of too much to do might have meant we'd like to shut off the phone, curl up on the couch, and put everything off for another day. After the Transition, Diane noticed that she wasn't feeling as overwhelmed anymore. She found herself ready to face challenges on the spot: starting a new project, having a tough conversation, speaking up or nipping a problem in the bud. "Yeah, that Scarlett O'Hara 'I'll think about it tomorrow' thing vanished after the Transition," Diane said.

"One thing that's happening," she told me, "is that I'm finding myself flustered in conversations with younger female colleagues. If one of them comes in with a rapid-fire stream of ideas, problems, and insights and wants my attention before I've finished what I'm working on, I lose it." Diane looked uncomfortable. "I don't want to make them feel bad. I want to support them. But it's hard to get them to take a breath, let me finish thinking through what they've said and not lose my train of thought on my own work."

Before the Transition, Diane might have done the same thing. Before the Transition, like most women, Diane would have been a rapid-fire multitasker.

Multitasking and anxiety go hand in hand. We don't know which comes first, but we do know they amplify each other. Doing too many things at once demands rapid switches of attention; that constant gear shifting might have given us a jolt of excitement over our own competence in our twenties and thirties, but now, during the Late Transition and the Upgrade, it makes the mind fuzzy, distracted, and unfocused. The key now is to calm the anxiety circuits that are triggered by multitasking so they don't set off another round of multitasking and anxiety. It can become a vicious cycle if we don't consciously intervene.

Many women who do learn to adjust to the Upgrade's new brain circuitry can experience a career boost, becoming better at each thing they do and more effective than they've ever been. Without the distractions of multitasking and the need to put things off, many reexperience a career momentum not felt since their twenties. That process of reenergizing is good for you on so many levels: Studies show that those with high career momentum in the Upgrade score better on measures of self-acceptance, independence, and effective functioning in our fifties and sixties, including stronger physical health.

Diane and I had a chance to talk about her frustration over losing the ability to multitask. "I feel like I'm losing my edge," she said, "and I don't want to stop working." I understood the feeling, but there's a reframe here that I have found very powerful in my own life. "What if," I responded, "you thought of it a bit differently? In the old days, doing a million things at once might have felt good at some level. But you and I both know from the science that we did everything less well as a result. Now your brain is demanding that you stay good and focused on one thing. You have a better chance of getting it right."

"So it might be a gift?"

"Yes, and not only for you, but if you're asking others to slow down as well, it can help them stay more focused and be more careful in their thinking. Your focus can act like a grounding wire for them."

Diane was pensive. Finally she said, "I'm starting to see how engaging my own brain's wiring can help me make better decisions. By going with the natural flow, I can allow the space for taking a good hard look at things, in a way I don't think I've ever given myself permission to do. This is true for my marriage, family, work, everything." By riding in the direction the horse was going, Diane was beginning to optimize her Upgrade.

Memory and Distractibility

Although the medical profession views the Transition and the Upgrade primarily as a reproductive transition, the impact is almost entirely neurological. Hot flashes, brain fog, anxiety, and sleep disruption indicate glitches in the pervasive estrogen-regulated nervous systems. In all human brains, including male, estrogen is a master regulator that works to ensure the brain gets its energy supply.

One of the neurological impacts of the decline of estrogen is change in memory function. By the time we have gone through the Transition, we have less estrogen in our brains than men—their testicles produce testosterone throughout their lives, and that converts to estrogen in the brain. Very low estrogen is hypothesized to be one reason women are more susceptible to dementia. And it's another infuriating inflection point for me: HT could likely have brain-protective benefits, and it looks like those benefits outweigh the risks pointed out in previous studies. It's been staring us in the face, but the doctors who shaped the research and the remedies missed it, focused as they have been on the body parts that interest the reproductive culture most. Hint: It's not our brains.

On the flip side, the impact of steady, lower estrogen on memory may have some psychological benefit. UCSF neurology professor Adam Gazzaley has done seminal work on memory and distractibility in the over-sixty female brain. What he discovered is that before the Transition, we could hold two things in mind, one in each hemisphere of the brain, and switch between the two channels by momentarily suppressing one and then switching back to the other. If you tried to hold a third thing, you would have to drop one of the other two. In the Upgrade, Gazzaley found, even a second thought cannot be suppressed and will knock the first one into the black hole of lost words and forgotten ideas. The two ideas collide in a bottleneck and one has to go. Just as the loss of collagen changes the structure of your skin, this is a normal structural change in how the brain works.

At first, not being able to hold more than one thing in the mind by switching back and forth can feel disconcerting. "I think I'm developing dementia," said Diane when she came to visit me over worries about memory. "My partner interrupted me and changed the subject. I got annoyed with him for doing it because I couldn't remember what I was about to say and I knew it was important. It took hours for the thought to come back." She looked visibly distressed.

I told her, and I'm telling you: That's not dementia. It's just normal. If you have one thing in your mind, a second idea will push the first one out and you won't be able to retrace to what the first one was. You just need a few work-arounds.

The hippocampus, prefrontal cortex, amygdala, neocortex, and cerebellum work in a beautiful choreography of laying down, while awake and asleep, short-term, long-term, emotional, and movement-coordination memory. A fight, a threat, or intense joy—any strong feeling—means the amygdala helps burn the details of an emotional memory into our minds forever. That's a memory we will retain. But if we were holding one thought when another enters, we will lose the original thought.

Dr. Gazzaley's work shows how the multitasking ability gets disrupted in the Upgrade. It's like this. You've got an email from a new friend with her phone number; you want to call her and have to input the number manually. You see the number, repeat it to yourself as you enter the digits. An alert pops up for an email that you click on. You might not only forget the phone number; you might forget that you wanted to call someone at all.

The brain's memory circuits in the Upgrade are forever changed, forcing us to newfound heights of focus. Because a new thought or interruption will knock the thing you were just about to do or say out of your short-term memory banks, you will learn to say, "Wait a minute. Let me just finish what I'm doing first." You must hold your ground in a new, forceful way so as not to lose your train of thought or momentum in your action.

Since I have an older husband, I have watched what he does. Here are some tips I've gleaned from watching him. The first is to schedule tasks according to the time of day when you have the best focus. The second is that as soon as you know you have to do something, jump on it right away and complete it. If you have to wait to do it, write it down in a place where you'll remember to read it. Sometimes I forget to read my reminder list, but that's another story. If you try to chase down a lost train of thought, you won't find it. You have to let it come back around on its own. It may be too late by the time it does, but that's just the new reality. You learn to let it go and giggle about it with friends.

Once Diane accepted that her brain network for memory had changed, she made a few adjustments. The first was that she relied on the emptier memory brain organs of younger colleagues. She started to warn younger colleagues about catching her in the hallway without her phone or her organizer. "They would stop me and tell me something on my way to the bathroom. By the time I got back to my desk, my mind was on something else," she said, "and I would have completely forgotten. I carried my phone and to-do list around more frequently, but if I didn't have it with me, I asked them to email me what they had just said, so that it would be at the top of my list when I got back to my desk. That worked."

My friend Kathryn turned distractibility into a communications superpower. Standing up to speak in front of a group used to scare her so badly in her thirties and forties that she was constantly battling her intestines for a long enough break from needing to go to the bathroom so that she could deliver her speech. Now, at sixty-five, she strides out onto the stage, faces 1,200 salespeople gathered for a conference on television ad sales, and barely looks at the ten words on the scrap of paper she's got tucked into her right hand. "I forget what I'm saying in the middle of a talk all the time. I lose my place, and instead of panicking, I ask the audience to help me. 'What was I saying?' or 'Now why am I talking about that?' I find they are not only willing to help, but they are excited that I've asked them to engage. And by the number of people who shout out reminders, I know whether or not I'm reaching them. If I'm not doing my job, they won't respond, or they'll give me the wrong answer. I spent decades in the bathroom freaking out about things like this when I was younger. If I made a mistake during a talk, I would pretend like nothing was wrong and white-knuckle it through the rest of the speech, hoping nothing else would go awry."

"When did everything change?" I asked.

"I was exhausted during a presentation. It was a really rough period—my career and first marriage were teetering on the brink—and I was rattled. I stopped to take a sip of water and spotted a friend in the audience whom I hadn't noticed earlier. We made eye contact and smiled. It was such a relief to see her face that I completely forgot where I was. I don't know what made me do it, but I blurted out what had just happened. All of it. That I had been nervous, super stressed about my life falling apart, and that seeing my friend made me feel so relieved I forgot what I was talking about. I was shocked when so many in the audience smiled and started helping me find my bearings. All those years I had thought they were waiting for me to fail. And now I could see they wanted me to succeed."

Memory and the Hamster Wheel of Worry

It seemed so benign, that coffee after breakfast. As she sat alone on a sunny day, looking out the kitchen window and just letting the mind wander, the memory of our conversation floated up in Kathryn's mind, she later told me. She smiled at her success and newfound ease. But that day, that month, that year, had been really bad, she thought. Then a flood of other memories: The couple who owned the business she worked for were fighting, and it was clear they were headed for a split. Kathryn's life was a daily hell of being put into positions of choosing sides. In the middle of that, she'd discovered some mysterious hotel credit card charges and had confronted her now-ex-husband. *How could you do this to us?* she remembered screaming at the top of her lungs as he confessed his affair. The entire fight was now in full bloom in her mind: the tired evening hours, the door slamming, the retreat to the guest bedroom, the sobbing, the lack of sleep. She thought of what she should have said instead of what was said, what she hoped to say if she saw him again. And those stepkids! She had put all her energy into them when their mother had checked out of their lives, and as soon as they heard their father was splitting with her, they blocked her. It was all as though it were happening in that moment, at breakfast, while sipping coffee. Living in these past and imagined future scenarios, she couldn't find her way to the present. She couldn't break the cycle. That's when she called me.

Kathryn was caught in rumination. Locked into the hamster wheel of worry, she'd lost her ability to be present, and that is a recipe for an unhappy brain state.

More than two thousand people signed up to participate in research on happiness conducted at Harvard in 2010 by two psychologists, Matthew Killingsworth and Daniel Gilbert. During the study, participants received text messages randomly throughout the day asking three simple questions: What are you doing? What are you thinking about? How happy are you feeling? Nearly half the time, people reported that their mind was wandering. And nearly all of the mind wanderers reported feeling much less happy than those who were focused on the task at hand. Those who responded that they felt connected to what they were doing in the moment reported being pretty happy.

Wild and unfettered, we let the mind and imagination go where it will. After school and work and raising families, this kind of freedom sounds like just the ticket to joy and happiness. Well, it turns out the opposite can be true. Just as children and teenagers crave structure or they become anxious and afraid, an unsupervised wandering adult mind quickly becomes unhappy. It doesn't mean you should spring into action and keep busy. Your brain will need the quiet. But unless you're a very experienced meditator, you'll need some tricks and tips for managing that quiet in order to make the new calm delicious.

Science has only recently discovered why, when the mind is left to daydream without a goal or direction, things tend to go negative pretty quickly. The key turns out to be the brain's default mode network (DMN), which was discovered in 1979. Part of the function of this system is to allow us to do familiar tasks like making the bed, fixing breakfast, and driving safely almost on autopilot. We repeat some things so often that the DMN incorporates them into its circuitry and we no longer have to think about what we are doing. Because the DMN is wired into the memory network, it uses what we know already, so that a thing we do or think about over and over again becomes effortless over time. It becomes a skill.

One of those skills is being alert to danger. It was super useful when humans lived in the wild: That alertness made sure we would see and remember places that could put the lives of ourselves and our tribe on the line.

Now that we are not living in the wild, you'd think that the danger vigilance would quiet a bit. Guess again. Even after millennia of living in increasingly safe times, the brain has turned this instinct into a full-on cognitive distortion called negativity bias. It acts as a filter and makes it feel realistic to be pessimistic, to look for problems where there are none.

As a result, if we leave the mind to its own devices, unsupervised daydreaming turns negative quickly. Our dreams of a happy and free mind turn unpleasant fast. When the mind is wandering, i.e., in default mode, the brain turns into that big ball of Velcro that rolls around picking up negative thoughts. Since the DMN is also connected to the long-term memory network, those negative thoughts will tend to be autobiographi-cal memories: Your worst, your scariest, your most depressing experiences jump to the front of the line, screaming like an eager, smart-ass kid in school, *Me! Me! Pick me! I know the answer!* And you will pick that eager negative thought almost every single time. The mind will get pulled, as if by a magnet, to worry, bad relationships, regrets about the past, big fears about the future. When memories and scenarios arise in full bloom, our wandering mind leads us not to joy; it gets sucked into the vortices of unhappiness, shame, guilt, anger. Everything will feel and look so much worse than it is. But at the time, we won't know that.

As Kathryn was discovering over her morning coffee, when the unsu-pervised mind is stuck in negative thoughts, memories, and scenarios, parts of the prefrontal cortex become locked into a pattern we experience as rumination. It's the hamster wheel of worry that sucks us into the downward spiral of agitation, fear, and sadness. Once the thought pattern starts, it feels as though you can't get off. And in 2020, researchers dis-covered why it's so hard to break out of rumination once it starts.

After priming research participants for moments of rumination by having them remember times of rejection, researchers observed brain activity in an fMRI. What they saw was as riveting as rumination itself: Two areas of the cortex, the TPJ (temporoparietal junction) and the precuneus, lit up in a robust, exclusive partnership. These two brain areas are part of the DMN. Their functions, having to do with memory, integration of information from the body and the environment, and perception of the environment, can hijack cognition into a feedback loop that becomes something akin to an unbreakable magnetic lock. When this brain-organ partnership is in control, we can start believing that all our thoughts are accurate and real, regardless of how crazy they might seem when faced with the truth. The mag-lock state of mind prevents new insights from entering; it disables creativity and innovation; it blocks us from being able to find new solutions to old problems. Remember, the cascade that led to the trap of rumination began with a wandering, daydreaming mind. When we start to believe the thoughts of failure, doom, and gloom, it can snap the tent pole in half.

Breaking the Rumination Mag Lock

The good news is that in the same 2020 study, researchers documented the effectiveness of cognitive techniques for breaking the magnetic lock of the TPJ and precuneus that are stuck in rumination. The techniques had to do with how we talk to ourselves, what we believe to be true about ourselves, and how we can put a setback or even a flaw into perspective.

On that sunny morning, Kathryn was stuck reliving the moment of her ex-husband's betrayal. She told me that along with rumination came labels: *I'm alone. I'm a failure at marriage. I must be unlovable if my husband would cheat on me. I'm a nasty, rageful person because I was ruthless in slicing his ego to the bone when I confronted him.* Soon these labels formed into solid beliefs that became difficult to shake; they became the bait that sucked her back into replaying and reimagining scenes again and again. To break the lock, I asked Kathryn if she was the only one who was ever betrayed, if she was the only one who wanted revenge when they were hurt, if no one ever recovered after an event like this, or if there might be a positive side to her rage, like not being intimidated easily and being able to speak up for herself. I asked her if there was any way to accept that it's okay to have negative emotions in difficult times and that having tough times is part of being human. And finally I asked her to consider that negative emotions and setbacks can be overcome. I asked her to give herself the time to think clearly about tiny steps she could take that, over days, weeks, and months, could form solutions. She agreed to spend ten minutes daily journaling about these possibilities.

This is called reframing. When participants' brains were scanned in the fMRI using the same kinds of reframing and reappraisal techniques I was suggesting to Kathryn, they were able to track the progress they were making in decoupling the mag lock of the TPJ and the precuneus. Forty percent of participants were successful in physically and emotionally emerging from the brain lock of rumination.

New interventions for the rumination that comes with depression will be found as a result of this work, and I believe it's going to show us what monks and meditators, and Gilbert and Killingsworth's 2010 Harvard study on focus, have already shown: that being present, focused on what we are doing, makes us happy, and that with the right tools and practice, we can make a difference in our brains, in the happiness in our minds, and make room for the joy in our lives. After I talked all of this through with Kathryn, she added to her morning ritual one minute of focusing on her breathing before beginning her reframing exercise in her journal.

When I first started digging into this subject, I was full of questions. Reappraisal and reframing have long been known to be effective interventions in cognitive behavioral therapy (CBT). They free us to think and see differently by helping us uncover and challenge distorted thoughts and feelings about who we are. Seeing the neuroscience behind how we can get stuck in ruminative distortions, going around and around about something in the past or an imagined future conflict, and learning how we can use that science to break out of the cycle is an illuminating first step.

Why do I say *first* step? Because smashing a ruminative cycle is a momentary intervention. This pull to negative thoughts is an ancient habit, deeply wired into the oldest parts of the human brain. Like a heavy smoker mindlessly picking up the next cigarette, we will go there again and again. In the Upgrade, I personally want my days, nights, thoughts, and emotions to be about comfort in my skin, quality connection with others, the ability to pursue my real passions. I want the clear mental and emotional bandwidth to imagine into the Upgrade, to use creativity to innovate in the second half of life. I want to see clearly the path toward manifesting purpose. If I'm trapped in rumination, I will be stuck repeating old patterns. And I didn't gain all of this wisdom and experience just to have it locked up by the magnetic pull of rumination.

I want to become skilled at prevention, skilled at working with attention, focus, and developing meta-awareness—alertness to patterns of thoughts, feelings, and emotions. It's an awareness that gives us the chance to catch the mind in the act of wandering, to stop it before it goes down a rabbit hole. It gives us the chance to change direction when imagination steers itself toward that magnetic dark place. Kathryn and I have been practicing these skills and talking about our experiences. It has helped us both stay on track.

Focus: The Steering Wheel of the Mind

There are a lot of potholes around San Francisco, and if I'm not careful when I drive there, my wheels get knocked out of alignment. When that happens, if I let go of the wheel for just a moment, the car will veer out of its lane. When we let go of the steering wheel of the mind, we let go of meta-awareness, awareness of what we are thinking and feeling right now. If we don't keep our hands on the wheel, we will veer out of the lane of well-being and straight into rumination.

The amount of worry, the type of worry, differs between the genders. Women worry more about safety, of others especially. Mothers constantly suppress ruminations about their children getting into accidents. That doesn't change as we get older. At ninety you worry about your seventy-year-old kid getting cancer. The echoes of mommy-brain wiring will produce these scenarios, these unsupervised daydreams. These negative scenarios lead to fixation, but that isn't focus; it's just the mag lock of rumination. Fixation is part and parcel of the hamster wheel of negative thought. It's the rigidity of obsession over a person, a substance, an object, or status. It's the earworm you can't get out of your mind that replays a song in your head for hours.

Focus is flexible, allowing you to notice when you're headed off into fixation, stop, and bring the mind back to the present. It's the opposite of unsupervised daydreaming, the wandering default-mode mind. It sounds awkward and self-conscious to stay alert and aware, like having to constantly chase a rambunctious toddler. But once upon a time, putting a spoon to your mouth, brushing your teeth, riding a bike, driving a car, all were awkward, self-conscious affairs. Over time, those skills were transferred into the DMN, the same network responsible for the wandering, ruminating, perseverating mind. As a new habit was practiced, as coordination and muscles became stronger, those activities became automatic. A lightly focused, relaxed, ready, clear, alert, and aware mind can also become a habit. As the activity of lightly steering the mind becomes habit, it can be transferred to the DMN. Over time (and I don't mean days, weeks, or months; we are talking years) it too becomes effortless. Without the waves of monthly hormone cycles pushing and pulling at the brain's circuitry, focus gets easier.

Like a squirmy toddler told to sit still, attention will wander off the minute you try to gently rest it on anything. It's what minds do. We can either get frustrated or enjoy its energy and creativity. The act of bringing the mind back from wandering, or fuzziness if you get sleepy, is what makes us stronger. Like repeated bicep curls, it's how muscles develop.

We can use new muscles of awareness to keep from going down the usual what-if rabbit holes of worry, negative comparisons to others, unrealistic expectations, and belief that our fears about the future are true. In the Upgrade it is our job to find better alternatives to the mind being triggered into negative wandering: shutting off social media, going for a walk, using the Breathe app on our iPhone or Apple Watch, saying no to a call or lunch with a toxic person.

For those who have an overactive mind or a mind that won't sit still, sometimes movement or stretching first helps. For Kathryn, images of balance helped. "I have always had a hard time settling down," she said, "and it got more intense during the Transition. Concentration was really hard. The only time I could focus was while doing balancing poses in yoga." It makes sense: There's a lot at stake, maybe even broken bones if you fall, so the cerebellum activates the network necessary for alertness to balance. You can leverage the same neurocircuitry by conjuring the feeling of trying to balance on a stability disk, a beam, whatever works, to recruit the alertness of balancing the mind on the present moment or an object or subject—like a nurturing moment (see appendix, page 258), safety, relaxation, or compassion—of meditation.

The brain in meditation kicks up the best of the nervous system and neurochemicals. Oxytocin and dopamine, bonding, and reward chemicals are released. Anytime you focus on the breath, the vagal system is activated. Steadying your attention on the breath signals the vagus nerve to activate the relaxing parasympathetic nervous system, counteracting the sympathetic nervous system—the threat-response system that is fired up by the adrenals. A nurturing moment signals safety and prepares the vagus nerve to stimulate the parasympathetic system.

Alternate-nostril breathing, watching the breath, body scan, present-moment awareness, prayer, the nurturing moment, compassion training, twelve-step programs (see appendix, pages 251 and 257). There are so many methods, and you've likely heard or seen them or been guided through one during a yoga class. If you take nothing else away from this, I want you to remember that focus holds the key to the Upgrade. If you can learn and practice a method for very brief periods daily and eventually without being guided, you will start to be able to take the wheel of your own mind and steer it happily in the direction you'd like to go. You can start with just thirty seconds. That's the Dalai Lama's recommendation.

The opposite of the perseverating mind is one that is motivated by something that brings it lasting joy: Diane's rediscovered focus at work;

Alina's new passion for the environment; Kathryn's harnessing of her mind; my excitement about the Upgrade. Imagining, manifesting, and stabilizing our own Upgrade becomes a choice. The best news is that the quieting of hormonal waves puts the focus we need more within our reach. It gets easier to choose.

Life Span or Health Span

Chapter 14

My mother's friend Belle divorced in the 1940s and never remarried. An avid golfer and outdoor enthusiast, she went on safari alone in the fifties. She had lovers in Australia and Italy. She never used a golf cart; she loved walking the course. When she reached her eighties, she opted for playing nine holes over getting a lift.

She was sharp as a tack and never turned the volume down on her New York voice. Grandchildren giggled as they held up the handset of the old touch-tone phone for others to hear across the room. She read avidly, played a weekly bridge game, and indulged in a sip of sherry after dinner until the day she died at eighty-four. Though she wasn't ill, she was climbing the stairs to her doctor's office for a checkup when she got tired and sat down on the steps, and her heart gave out.

My great-aunt Harriett, who was married to a difficult man with a sometimes violent temper, lived until she was ninety-five. She didn't exercise most of her life, including after her husband died, when she was in her late sixties. She was a heavy martini drinker and didn't much worry about what she was putting into her body, other than the concern over what might make her gain weight. Her cognitive decline began in her early seventies—it was clear to her family she had been struggling with her hearing for a decade, but she refused to do anything about it. Hearing loss and cognitive decline can come together. No one is sure if hearing aids stop its progress, but we are sure that they decrease the chance of depression from isolation; depression does impact our ability to think clearly and regulate emotions. The family had good reason to worry about the fact that Harriett was too proud for hearing aids.

Harriett's knees gave out and she stopped being able to travel by the time she turned eighty, remaining homebound and mostly alone other than frequent trips to the doctor to keep adjusting her increasing list of medications for blood pressure, fear and sadness, joint pain, and insomnia. She spent the last seven years of her life with full-time care, her mind ravaged by Parkinson's. Unable to recognize her family members, her emotions were in a constant state of turmoil. She suffered until the end.

Harriett's life span was eleven years longer than Belle's. But her health span, that period of time in which she was able to enjoy a quality of life that included both physical and mental energy, was perhaps fourteen years shorter. Everyone would like to exercise their own preference for how they want to live; in the Upgrade, personally, I choose health span over life span. But how available is that choice?

Measuring Medical Success

Think for a minute about how success in medicine is measured. There is one marker: whether or not a patient dies. Success is not measured by quality of health or life of the person who doesn't die. Success could mean someone is bedridden or in a lifelong coma. When avoiding death is the only marker for success, what does that mean for quality of life?

For more than one hundred years, medicine's single-pointed focus on increasing life span has resulted in world-changing innovations powered by the young men, and a few women, who set out on the noble mission of saving lives. We have penicillin; vaccines for smallpox, polio, pneumonia, and COVID-19; heart medications; chemotherapy for cancer; organ transplants; cholesterol-lowering medications; artificial joints. All of these medicines and protocols support life; and in focusing on cancer and cardiovascular health, we have bent the curve on early death. That's a great thing. Yet at the same time it has come at a huge cost.

America now has the biggest and most expensive medical system in the world. Residents spend more on "healthcare" than any other nation in the world, and so it would seem that those who live in the United States would have a longer life span and better health outcomes than everyone else. But it isn't true. When you compare the life span and health of Americans to those of residents of all other developed nations, the United States has the worst outcomes in nearly every category, including longevity, heart disease, cancer, and especially maternal and infant mortality.

Women in the second half are bound to fare a bit worse in terms of health span, though we don't have any way of knowing directly, since the data have never been collected. But it's not hard to extrapolate; women's health, other than reproductive health, has barely been part of the equation in medical education. It's been ignored that women over sixty are the fastest-growing demographic in suicides, even though the numbers are right there staring us all in the face. Yet with all of these unfavorable outcomes, young doctors who see defeating death as the central goal of research and practice continue to set the agenda not just for medicine but for the quality of our lives as we age.

Knowledge May or May Not Be Power

We can't control every factor that impacts our health span. There are a vast number of factors and circumstances that can cause illness. It's impossible to account or control for everything. Poverty can increase our risk for heart and respiratory disease; so can our mother's smoking while pregnant with us. Trauma has an impact on life span as well as disease susceptibility, and we can be unknowingly poisoned by what's in the air, water, or soil around us. Those who grew up in a certain area of New Jersey have a higher risk for bladder cancer because of toxins in the water.

Those who grew up around the Gulf Coast's Golden Triangle area, where oil is refined, have a higher risk for asthma and blood cancers. The death of a child or spouse can lead to broken-heart syndrome, impacting our health. None of these things is our fault. We are not losers, nor is anyone else, because of being affected by circumstances beyond our control, because of the suffering that is inevitably part of the human condition. That life itself always ends in death is not a mistake; it is reality.

Genetics do play a role that is also beyond our control. Nancy Wexler is a renowned geneticist who devoted her career to studying the gene for Huntington's disease, a debilitating and fatal hereditary condition that runs in her family. If you have one parent who carries the gene, there is a fifty-fifty chance you will get it. It is what we call a single-gene dominant inheritance disorder: If the one gene is present, the chance of developing Huntington's is 100 percent. Dr. Wexler's mother died of the disease; it took the lives of her uncles and her grandfather as well. And she inherited it too.

There are many conditions for which we can detect genetic causes. The BRCA mutation for breast cancer; the APOE4 variant for Alzheimer's; the sickle cell gene for sickle cell disease. Not every mutation means that a gene gets expressed. With Huntington's, we know that it does, and the same is true for those who carry two copies of sickle cell mutation. One hundred percent of those who carry two sickle cell gene mutations will get sick. But with others, just because you have the gene doesn't mean you will get the disease. With the BRCA gene, up to 80 percent of the women with this mutation will develop breast cancer, but not everyone. Even two APOE4 variants don't inexorably lead to Alzheimer's disease in all cases.

When you have a family history of a disease, there is a higher likelihood that you are carrying some of the relevant genes, and there are some disorders, such as breast cancer, in which we already have DNA tests that can inform you about your relative risk. Whether or not you want to get that information is a deeply personal decision. Sometimes knowing can mean you have the chance to engage in preventive activities, like more vigilance with diagnostic technology or even prophylactic mastectomy and ovariectomy if you have the BRCA mutation. You can also learn if a certain kind of chemotherapy is likely to work on a particular cancer based on your own genetic makeup. So genetic information can in some cases guide a course of action. In many cases, genetic information has no practical actionable value. And don't expect it to tell you what you should be eating. The testing just isn't that sophisticated yet.

What we learn from doctors and genetics can feel like destiny and cause us to make life-altering decisions. Rachel Naomi Remen, the author of *Kitchen Table Wisdom,* was told at a young age that her severe Crohn's disease would shorten her life. The doctors informed her that she wouldn't live past forty. As a result, she chose not to marry or have children, because she didn't want to inflict the suffering of losing a wife or mother on a family. But she didn't die at forty. She's in her eighties as of this writing.

How Remen's life would have been different if she had not been informed of a likely early death is impossible to know. But there is some evidence that could make an argument for not knowing. There is a category of older people whom medicine has labeled super-agers. These are people in their seventies, eighties, and beyond whose mental acuity and physical activity reflect the age of someone decades younger. As part of a study in Southern California, the brains of some super-agers were scanned after their deaths. In the cases of several women in their nineties who had been active physically up until the end, engaged in things like a weekly bridge game, researchers were shocked by their MRI scans: Their brains showed the same kind of moth-eaten appearance as the brains of some Alzheimer's patients. And when their brains were dissected after death, they were full of the tangles and plaques of typical Alzheimer's patients— yet their minds were cognitively intact. No one ever told them that they had scans that should reflect extreme cognitive decline. The question I have is how the knowledge of these brain scans might have impacted the way these super-agers lived. Would they have remained super-agers, or would they have given up if they had been told by a doctor that their scans were showing strong signs of dementia? Would they have been given medicines whose side effects might have decreased their quality of life or set off more cognitive decline?

There is in medicine something we call "incidental findings." In my midforties I kept spraining my ankle. Orthopedists did repeated X-rays, and not finding anything, they put me in orthotics. When that didn't work, I was sent for an MRI. This time they found a disease: osteochondritis dissecans, which means "a hole in the ankle bone." The doctors decided that this hole in my ankle was the cause of all my trouble. But when I learned that fixing that hole could end up creating more trouble, I decided to work with a physical therapist instead. While doing some massage, the therapist released some tendon and muscle contractions that were pulling my ankle in a funny direction. Within six months the problem was fixed. Twenty years later, I haven't had another sprained ankle.

The hole in my bone had nothing to do with the problem in my ankle. It was an "incidental finding." Sometimes a finding is a red herring, and doctors will end up telling a story about it that isn't really the story. Not every finding in a scan is the direct cause of a complaint. It might or might not be.

Nancy Wexler opted not to have the genetic test for Huntington's. If she discovered too young that she carried the gene, she felt it would disempower her from living a full life. So she decided to live as healthy and vigorous a life as possible. By her early seventies, she had become fairly debilitated by the symptoms of Huntington's, but she told me she didn't regret her decision for a minute.

This is not to say that ignorance is always bliss. But you can make a discerning choice about how information may impact your decision making. Doctors have noted that people "die on time"; when told they are expected to have a certain period of time to live, they tend to live exactly that amount of time. Because it happens so frequently, many medical professionals have begun to think this is not just because they are such good prognosticators. The power of suggestion is huge. If you are going down the road of genetic testing, find a doctor and genetic counselor who will take the time to really explore options. Get multiple opinions and perspectives. This is not a one-stop internet shopping moment.

Since my Transition, I am clear about how I want to age and that health span is my marker for success. I want my mind to be sharp and my body to be mobile. I know I don't have total control over all the factors that go into how I age, but there are things available to me that I can do to make sure I do my best to remain cognitively sharp, fearless, active, and as energetic as I can be. There's no guarantee that if I do everything right I will end up with the perfect outcome. Anything can happen. But how I emerge into the later decades of the Upgrade can be shaped by what I do now.

Our Real Risks: Cognitive Decline and Alzheimer's

Cancer is so mysterious. In its early forms it's painless, and you might only feel a lump or find it on a scan. As a medical student, while reading about the disease, I kept feeling my abdomen and breasts a couple of times a day, looking for signs of painless lumps. The more I read, the more I checked. In those days I didn't know what fibrocystic or lumpy breasts were, but I had them; I thought every bump was breast cancer and that I was a goner. It wasn't true. Reading about a disease makes us suggestible, and it's a common phenomenon among medical students that we become sure we have what we are reading about.

Women have some real risks for Alzheimer's, but it doesn't mean you will get it. I don't want you to have to go through what I went through as a med student, thinking you have a disease you are learning about. So while absorbing the following, remember the super-agers, who were in full control of cognition into their nineties even though their brain scans looked like they should have had dementia. Remember Belle walking the golf course and playing bridge. Remember normal structural changes to the brain that keep us from multitasking in the Upgrade. Keep all of this in mind as you read the next section, and maybe it will help keep you from getting stuck on the hamster wheel of worry.

While women on average are more resilient to cognitive decline and memory loss that comes with age, one-fifth of all women will be diagnosed with Alzheimer's disease (AD). As with cancer and heart disease in the 1950s, we don't have good treatment options. The most common form of dementia is AD, and the risk for AD is higher in women than in men. The biggest reason appears to be that women live longer. Both sexes show a similar risk of developing AD until advanced ages—in the eighties, when women show increased risk, one in five women versus one in ten men. But the theory is that by the time people reach their eighties, the less hardy men have already died off. If more of them had survived, researchers assume that they'd be at equal risk.

With all the brain benefits of estrogen, there's been a lot of speculation about a possible role in prevention of AD. But multiple studies have shown that starting estrogen after the age of sixty doesn't help. And in 2003 a large study on women who carried at least one APOE4 variant showed that starting estrogen plus progestin after the age of sixty-four was associated with an increase in dementia. While we know that estrogen is good for memory and learning, starting it at the wrong time can be more harmful than helpful. So if you're more than ten years past the Upgrade and haven't started HT, it's probably better not to. But if you are between forty-five and fifty-five, studies suggest that taking HT long-term may reduce your risk of getting any neurodegenerative disease, including Alzheimer's. Remember that all the other strategies—self-care, movement, sleep, diet, stress modulation, care for the microbiome—will have a positive impact on preservation of cognition.

And while estrogen on its own hasn't been shown to treat Alzheimer's, estrogen does have proven brain benefits. HT sets the brain up for helping you take action against inflammation that might speed cognitive decline. The growth in the brain stimulated by estrogen brings a more positive outlook, an enthusiasm for life, and energy for motivation to engage in self-care. All of this helps preserve cognition. Studies have shown that women who carried the APOE4 variant but engaged in moderate cardio for five to six hours per week and kept cholesterol low with a better diet and statins preserved cognition for a longer period.

If you are among the 2 to 3 percent of the population that carries two APOE4 variants, you may have up to a 90 percent chance of developing Alzheimer's. And for the 25 percent of women who carry one APOE4 the risk is higher too. But keep in mind that only 37 percent of those who have AD have the APOE4 variant. And for many of us the risk is less. So whatever your risks, there are things you can do to mitigate the odds. As soon as you realize you are in the Mid- or Late Transition, exercise, stop smoking and drinking alcohol, and keep your weight and cholesterol under control. Discuss taking HT with your doctor. The impact on inflammation in the brain and on protecting cognition is well documented for each of these strategies. Do them all together if you can.

Puppies. Kittens. Babies. Hug one or find a video to get your oxytocin going. Then breathe to stop the spiral into ruminative certainty that you have Alzheimer's. There's a very good chance you don't. But since women have a higher risk for it, I want you to know the reality.

Here's the case for HT and brain health. Estrogen is essential to a cascade of neurochemical processes in the brain. It helps neurons connect. It helps the brain use glucose, sugars, for energy. It helps the immune system protect neurons from harm, strengthening the brain's ability to bounce back from inevitable assaults like inflammation and to find its balance again. It kicks off a bunch of feel-good reactions, including production of GABA, the antianxiety neurochemical, and the release of endorphins, like those we get from a runner's high, which soothe pain and depression. Estrogen is beneficial to circulation, and in the brain that means a good strong flow of blood, oxygen, and nutrients to keep it healthy. Estrogen helps regulate inflammation in the brain, which means that those astrocytes and microglia have a chance to perform their function of cleaning out the trash and feeding the brain cells, more so in female brains than male. Regulation of inflammation means a lower chance of microglia and astrocytes going into zombie mode, spewing toxins and further endangering cognition. This may be one reason that women in their forties, who still have estrogen, are less likely to get early onset Alzheimer's than men of the same age.

The Early- to Mid-Transition is a shock to the brain and the circuits in the female brain change quite a lot compared with those of men of the same age. The bottoming out of estrogen causes sudden crashes in brain energy. This inhibits the brain's ability to access its usual source of energy and use that energy efficiently. Estrogen is the master regulator of metabolism in the female brain and promotes glucose uptake—glucose is the brain's favorite fuel. Estrogen dials up the energy of mitochondria, the powerhouse of all cells in the body. It protects cells from the damage caused by toxins emitted by aging cells; it prevents cell death; and it helps balance calcium in the body and builds strong bones. It helps keep the blood-brain barrier healthy, preventing damaging substances circulating in the blood from getting into the brain. The role of estrogen in the brain is the same for men, but they never experience the Transition, this sudden hormone drop, the accompanying loss of gray matter and white matter, or wholesale remodeling of brain circuits. Testosterone converts into estrogen, and so they have a fairly continuous lifetime supply. Some scientists are now investigating if the loss of estrogen for women in the Transition is a tipping point for cognitive decline.

The drop in estrogen means the mechanism for transporting glucose through the blood-brain barrier is dramatically diminished, triggering a cascade of metabolic effects as the brain tries to adjust to lower levels of glucose. It means that proinflammatory cytokines in the brain are less well regulated. Lower estrogen is why we have hot flashes, why we become more likely to develop diabetes, and why inflammation becomes less easily managed. "I was surprised," Terri told me, "that after lifelong perfect blood work, my inflammatory markers skyrocketed during the Transition. I couldn't absorb why that was happening, and nobody told me it was because of my hormone changes."

The brain fog that comes with the Transition and Early Upgrade is not dementia, and it's not presaging Alzheimer's disease. Its cause and cure is estrogen. The brain fog is a result of lower estrogen, and it can be fixed through HT. I repeat: It's not dementia. It's not the onset of dementia. It's temporary and fixable.

It's the reason I had my surgeon slap an estrogen patch on my butt in the recovery room after my total hysterectomy in 2005. Even while conventional medical wisdom was terrified by that 2002 WHI report warning of the dangers of HT, I knew the report was flawed and decided my brain health outweighed the risks.

This was my personal choice. Yours may be different.

If you decide not to take HT, or if it's contraindicated, do everything you can to fight inflammation: move, eat right, sleep well, destress wherever you can. You'll find some plans in the appendix.

Many women, knowing they have a family history of Alzheimer's or knowing they have one or two APOE4 variants, are getting baseline brain scans to track what they might feel is an inevitable slide into dementia. For me personally, knowing what I know about super-agers, I question whether or not it's information I would want to have. If the information indicated a course of action, then, yes, I would want it. But with APOE4 status? The only thing I could do to reduce my risk would be to engage in habits that reduced inflammation and take a statin so that the brain didn't decay quite as quickly. It turns out that statins reduce risk of dementia by almost 30 percent. And that's why I'm doing everything I can—focus, meditation, food, controlling cholesterol, movement, sleep, social connection, calm—to keep my brain in the Upgrade.

I'm afraid that if I knew I had the APOE4 variant, I'd be a wreck, constantly reading the tea leaves for signs that my disease had begun. But that's not true for everyone. I'd become obsessive about it. For Paula Spencer Scott, author of *Surviving Alzheimer's*, knowing her APOE4 status gave her power. Instead of causing her stress and depression, as some researchers feared, it motivated her to get a complete workup. When she saw that some of her inflammation markers were high and learned that these could cause a more rapid decline in brain health, it motivated her to act. She writes:

There's nothing like proof of weakness to motivate behavior change. For the first time in my life, I joined a gym and hired a trainer and began brain-beneficial high-intensity interval training.

(Just walking—my old exercise—wasn't enough, I learned.) I became even more vigilant about my Mediterranean diet, took prescribed supplements, learned "brain breaks" like mindfulness and more.

Two years on, my improved cognitive scores and lower cholesterol keep me going. As does finding myself in stronger shape at 60 than I was at 40. (True, I gained several pounds . . . but of muscle.)

I now run every choice I make through the lens of my brain health: *Is this helping or harming?*

For someone else, testing might raise urgency about lousy sleep, hypertension, poor glucose control, or stress. Swiss researchers have suggested that having motivational reserve—motivation to improve one's cognitive health—may even have a protective effect on the course of mild cognitive impairment.

The Hidden Brain Dangers of OTC and Prescription Drugs

Carole was beside herself. "Louann, my mom has gone downhill so quickly, and I just don't understand it," she said, on the edge of tears. "She's been in great shape—exercising, super active, and super sharp. I don't know what's going on. In less than two weeks she went from totally independent to needing full-time care. She's completely disoriented."

I had met Carole's mother, Helen. She was in her early eighties and didn't have genetic risks for Alzheimer's. Carole's grandmother had lived into her nineties and had her cognitive powers until the end. I asked if we could all get together and if Carole could collect any over-the-counter and prescription drugs her mother was taking.

We sat down in the living room, and on the coffee table was the answer. Her bottles of pills were all laid out, and there in full view was a bottle of nortriptyline. It is a tricyclic antidepressant being used in many pain clinics, and it had been prescribed two weeks earlier for chronic arthritic pain. It can cause dry mouth, dry eyes, and difficulty urinating. If drying up and trouble controlling functions is happening in one part of your body, it's happening also in your brain. For some people, this effect of anticholinergics can deliver a wallop to focus, memory, concentration, the entire memory system, as an anticholinergic. Remember, choline and acetylcholine are neurochemicals that govern the wake/sleep cycle and are part of the neurochemical process involved in memory consolidation. Tylenol and Benadryl also have anticholinergic effects.

Not everyone has side effects from nortriptyline, but as we age, side effects become more likely. When you hit seventy-five, due to a decrease in metabolism, it takes longer for the body to clear a drug. At age fifty, you might have been able to metabolize Valium in twenty-four hours, but at seventy-five, it could still be in your body three to ten days later. When patients continue to take it every day, the buildup gets too high and they can exhibit signs of dementia.

Once-a-day dosing of drugs is based on the average metabolism of twenty-to-fifty-year-old males. All pediatricians know you have to adjust doses for children to levels that are based on their body weight and metabolism. But it's not always done for small women and people over the age of fifty. Not even for those over seventy-five, whose body weight and muscle mass have gone down, taking their metabolism down too. With decreased metabolism, the half-lives of drugs, the time it takes for the body to clear them, becomes longer. This applies to supplements too. It's not inconceivable that effective doses of certain drugs could mean taking them once a week.

If a patient is in good communication with the doc, the doc will lower the dose. But with memory problems, confusion, or emotional issues, usually we will think, *It's just me. I'm getting old, and this is what happens.* But if family, friends, spouses, and doctors are smart about this and can get a patient off the meds, things can turn around immediately. Getting Helen off the nortriptyline cleared her cognitive problems within a few days. Anticholinergic drugs are a well-known *reversible* cause of memory problems.

The decision to take something preventively has to be driven by knowing that it will be more beneficial than harmful. More women are harmed by bleeding stomach ulcers caused by daily baby aspirin than are prevented from having strokes. Not only that, but daily baby aspirin can cause the very effect we might take it to prevent. If you already have plaques and you're taking aspirin or a blood thinner, you can develop little hemorrhagic bleeds in the arterial plaques. Those plaques then come loose and can cause a stroke—the very thing you're taking aspirin or a blood thinner to prevent. That's why the recommendation was finally dropped, especially for women. If you are in a high-risk group for heart disease, then taking something for prevention or taking an action to reverse the risk is the right thing to do. If you are having a heart attack, call 9-1-1, and immediately chew a full-sized regular aspirin. If you are at low risk, prevention may not only be useless but might be harmful. If you're in a moderate-risk zone, it's a question mark. Discuss with your doctor.

There have been a lot of heart attacks in my family. I had slightly elevated LDL (bad cholesterol), and my blood pressure was borderline high at 130/80, and so in my early sixties I wanted to see if I was also at risk of a heart attack. I had a sophisticated scan to see if I had calcium buildup indicating the possibility of plaque formation. I was in the 56 percent calcium range, and so my doctor put me on a statin called Crestor. Within a few days I developed blurred vision and brain fog. I couldn't function on the drug. So I asked, "Am I at high risk of heart attack?" The answer was "no." I probed further about her reasons for prescribing the drug. She began her sentence with "Studies show . . ." I stopped her there. Studies show lots of things, and the science constantly changes. I interrupted and said, "Okay, I've got to get off this statin." She said, "Fine. Let's follow up with more detailed tests and plan to check in every six months and monitor the situation." Since my LDL stayed high, I have followed the course of action and tried another statin. For now, we are trying to find one I can take. At the same time, I switched my estrogen from oral to topical. With oral estrogen, there is an increased risk of stroke. But that risk goes away with topical application, so I started using the patch again.

There is nothing that can replace the advice of a doctor you know and trust, so please don't mistake this for my telling you to get off your medications or to start HT. Your personal physician, *in partnership with* **you**, will know better. But do ask questions. Review all your medications and supplement dosages every year, and drop what you don't need. And take an advocate with you if your doctor is under fifty. The doctor may not hear your voice, and you'll need backup.

———

We need new markers for success to help shift the core values of medicine. We need to add quality-of-life markers, but until we can talk about death openly, as a reality, not a mistake, this conversation won't happen. Facing death, talking about it, may go against the nervous system's survival instinct, but not facing it means that we are all dealing with a persistent underlying anxiety caused by denial.

The best way to establish these markers comes from knowing what you want the biggest end point of all to look like for you. Communicating that verbally, and in writing, to your loved ones can open so many doors.

So Many Transitions

Chapter 15

I'm not Catholic, but my friend Diane convinced me to attend a ceremony in Washington, DC, for a cohort of novitiates who, after eleven
years of training, would take their full nun's vows. Seated near the back
of the cathedral, we watched as, one by one, dozens of bishops and cardinals processed toward the altar in towering scarlet hats making them
look eight feet tall. Censers swinging, organ playing, each took a velvet-
covered seat on the platform in the nave. I had never been to anything
like this—I grew up in a politically progressive Protestant church—and I
found it deeply uncomfortable. I felt the oppression of thousands of years
of male power in that moment.

The procession of bishops ended and then things got very quiet, very
still. It was similar to that moment of anticipation at a wedding, when the
atmosphere and music shift, cueing participants to turn for the bride's
entrance. I did not expect to experience what came next. A tiny woman,
barely five feet tall, stood in the doorway, illuminating the entire church
with her power, miniaturizing the posturing and pomp that had come
before. Mother Teresa walked slowly, smiling in her simple blue-and-
white sari, toward the altar and took her seat at the front left corner next
to several cardinals. She radiated peace. It was palpable. Her presence

transformed the cathedral atmosphere from rigidly ceremonious into un-contrived love and communion. I had never felt that kind of power ema-nate from a human being before, much less a woman.

Looking back, I see that Mother Teresa was manifesting her Upgrade. I don't have any illusions of becoming a saint, nor would I want to be. I didn't often agree with Mother Teresa's politics, but her love and service were undeniable. She was indefatigable. She never stopped caring or giv-ing. She didn't retreat to a slower, cozier, or more comfortable life. She never retired, seemingly impervious to society's unspoken axiom that at a certain age women are repulsive and have nothing left to offer.

Everything I've learned about the female brain and neurobiology has shown me that we women have been leaving our gifts at the door of the second half of life. It took me a long time to realize that giving in to that feeling, *I'm done; it's time to be cozy,* while comfortable, might not be an Upgrade. Instead, it might be a trap that leads to suffering as feelings of uselessness grow. It might cause suffering for generations of women who aren't being benefited by what we know. Escape into that kind of ease leaves future generations in the lurch to struggle for what we've failed to gain.

By the time women are over fifty, we've figured out a lot of things and we've accumulated wounds we've gone numb to (until our adult kids re-mind us of them). It's time to have a heart to heart with ourselves about being heard. "Before I got help with HT," said Terri, "I felt like I'd hit a wall. I kept waiting for the clarity and energy to come back so that I could take on complex, intense design projects again. I started to feel like I wasn't living a useful life anymore." I had a similar experience when I came up against the start-up energy of the very young. At their pace, I couldn't figure out what I had to offer. They had hired me for my thirty years of experience but didn't seem to slow down long enough to benefit from it. Our society doesn't honor wisdom, and so we tend not to honor the wisdom in ourselves. It took me a while to get comfortable with the difference in pace and to find my place in helping them see the big pic-ture.

Younger people convince themselves, and you, that they are the ones who have it together, and they are shocked when you see around corners they don't even know exist. It can take them a while to recognize what you have to offer, and they won't until we recognize that our time on the planet is a gift to them. In the same way we trusted our robust engagement in our twenties, we must continue to trust ourselves that we will find the place that lets us stand in the center of our authenticity. If we don't trust it now, when will we trust it?

Avoiding the cozy post-Transition trap and stepping into our own authority is a developmental phase of the second half of life, a phase that isn't mapped or charted or spoken about. It's one in which we refuse to agree that seeing women over fifty in an underwear commercial is disgusting. It's a developmental phase in which we don't quit because others are talking over us; we simply outlast them.

Genius is evenly distributed throughout society, regardless of race, gender, zip code, or gray hair dyed purple. We have too much to contribute to step off the stage now, when the world needs our wisdom, the wisdom of those who have put so much energy into solving problems for the preservation of life.

In psychology and psychiatry, we map developmental stages because it helps us contextualize someone's mindset so that we can better be of help. Common sense tells us that we can't use the same words or the same psychology for a fifteen-year-old boy as for a forty-eight-year-old woman. Each phase brings different challenges and has different goals. The burgeoning drive for independence in puberty can be a source of conflict in the family. As we grow into early adulthood, dreams of the future take hold and the prefrontal cortex is absorbed in running scenarios for building family, career, achievement, accumulation. Life during the fertility phase is lived in the future; psychologists have well mapped the developmental stage of so-called adulthood. But what are the stages like when there is no more runway for the future? Where does the imagination go and what are the new dreams? What are the problems to be solved between the end of the fertility phase and the end of life?

The Upgrade is a complete expression of the developmental stages of the second half of life. And to make the Upgrade possible, we need to know what the developmental stages are.

Defeating Transition Mind, Stage 1: Winning the Battle with the Demon of Appearance

It is sudden and disorienting when it happens in childhood, the moodiness and awkwardness that come with awakening sexuality. Over the years we learn how to inhabit this new identity. If we don't, the dissonance is enormous: The personality and outlook of a nine-year-old girl in a twenty-five-year-old body might get that woman sent straight to my office for help integrating and growing up, if it's not the result of a disorder about which nothing can be done.

There is a similar shift in sexual identity in the Transition and Early Upgrade. For the first time since puberty, our identity as sexual beings might feel as though it is beginning to crack. It's a shock to the system when we start to see that we no longer inhabit men's fantasies. It's hard to resist the pull of the insula wanting us to feel the way we are used to feeling in our own skin. It's hard to resist the demands of the insula to maintain that old identity through any means possible, including the brutally surgical. Yet just as it's disturbing to see a sexualized child or a childlike woman, there is a similar dissonance in seeing women try to inhabit an old identity in a new body and mind. It is exhausting to try to keep up an old appearance, holding reality at bay. And the people around you will feel uncomfortable. They won't tell you what they are feeling. They will instead exclaim wholeheartedly that the steps you've taken to prop up the old identity look great. The strong modulation in their tone of voice is often a compensation for shock, because the falseness can be alarming. They may take on a similar tone when we let our hair go gray and our skin wrinkle. At this stage of life, women can't win for losing.

As the natural preoccupation of our reproductive years, thinking about hair, makeup, clothes, body, and weight took up a lot of our daydreaming bandwidth. When I was younger, I remember that a new haircut or hair color often signaled—to both myself and others—that a new version of me was emerging. In the Upgrade, maybe that looks different; Instead of coloring my hair, maybe it's my natural color emerging. Instead of clothes that told the story of the sexy striver, maybe a new wardrobe and aesthetic tell more of the story of what's happening on the inside, one that reflects the quieting of those hormones. I find it deeply personal and quite scary to expose this internal process of Upgrading. I fear the reactions of my husband, family, friends, and enemies (especially!), that if I turn away from all that surgery, hair color, and cosmetics have to offer, they will find me gross. I fear being ostracized and humiliated, no longer invited to speak, to attend high-level conferences, to be in the center of the action, where I've spent most of my adult life. That reaction is normal. We are social beings as humans and particularly as females, so the idea of no longer belonging is, as you know by now, kryptonite to the female brain, even in the Upgrade. The fear of not belonging is one of the biggest obstacles to finding the courage to experiment with being myself at this age.

I'm still exploring a lot of this, but I've gotten this far: If my inside is kinder, friendlier, and less jealous, then I want my outside to more naturally reflect that I am no longer competing with other women for men or jobs. I want my outside to reflect competence, wisdom, and openness as opposed to sexiness and striving.

Knowing the power of the insula, I've made a conscious effort to combat its directives. I've had to think long and hard about what I want my appearance to say *now* about the inside of *me*, about how I want them to match up. It hasn't been a straightforward process. As I let go of the power of appearance, up pops the seemingly urgent feeling that if I want to stay in the game, I've got to look younger. I ask myself if I would still be taken seriously if I let my hair go white. And if the answer is "no," then do I adhere to the status quo or experiment with acts of rebellion that might move the needle for others? At the same time, I have yet to find a woman who has gray hair whom I think any less of. And so I ask myself to find the beauty in gray and to be honest about what game I'm trying to stay in. Regardless, it's a very personal decision.

It's a big adjustment in the early Upgrade to imagine and step into our new appearance. "My grandmother," Terri said, "was white haired and elegant. She wore simple, tailored clothes and very little makeup. Her bearing was regal. It was so natural to her that she didn't even know that's how people saw her. And that's what I want," she concluded, "though maybe a little updated with more athleisure and more comfortable shoes!" She's lucky to have had a role model.

Stage 2: Sex Becomes an Afterthought

How we feel about sex in the Upgrade is as much related to the demon of appearance as it is to the hormone shift that changes the reality of drive. It's another aspect of the same developmental shift that isn't mapped. "My body changed and I didn't feel sexy anymore," said Penny, fifty-three. "I didn't look good in sexy clothes, and it was hard to look at myself in the mirror." She had to spend time helping her brain and nervous system catch up to her new outer reality. But the inner reality was even more powerful.

After the Transition, when estrogen, oxytocin, and testosterone all go quiet, for many women, sexual reality shifts completely. It's as though the drive just evaporates. "When the symphony of intense bleeding finally came to a grand finale," said Penny, "I thought, *That's it? I don't have a sex drive?* It wasn't that I couldn't get my motor started. It's that I didn't even have a motor anymore. I had read enough to know that testosterone was the issue, and I begged my GYN to give me some. I was desperate not to lose my sex life. Until I got it, I had to trick myself into wanting sex," she said.

There was a moment in writing this book when I realized I had almost forgotten to write anything about sex. It's not that it hadn't been an important part of my life and relationship; of course it was. But one look at my testosterone levels, and those of many women in the Upgrade, tells the story of a reality shift, of a hunger that's gone away.

My friends Janet, fifty-five, and Sergio, sixty, had moved from New York to Argentina to Chicago and to three different homes in Dallas. Both had full-time jobs, but Janet ended up being project manager for every single move, even handling the Argentinian move in her broken Spanish. The evening after they made the second move within Dallas, she climbed into bed and told Sergio she was utterly exhausted, that she felt on the verge of a collapse. Without missing a beat, Sergio turned and asked her to help figure out the final plans for the electronics in the house. "My mind exploded," Janet said. "I looked at him and sobbed. Through the tears I said, 'I just told you I'm broken because of the move, and your response is to ask me to do something else for the house? To take on another project?'" Janet paused and, with a twinge of disbelief in her voice, she continued: "And then he capped it off by saying the best thing for me in that moment would be to have sex. Right then and there. As I was weak, and sobbing, and telling him I was broken. For the first time in more than a decade, I wanted to sleep in another room. I couldn't believe what I was hearing. Sex was the last thing I wanted, and it felt like another project I had to take on because it's what he wanted."

By the time we hit the Upgrade, unless we are taking supplemental testosterone, ours is up to three times lower than it was during our fertile years. It's not that we won't ever want sex again. It's more like not being hungry, yet still opening the refrigerator door to get something to eat just because it's dinnertime. The incredibly rich flourless chocolate torte you once craved with your whole being just doesn't seem as appealing. Okay, that's never happened to me, but you know what I mean.

Of all the women I've talked to, many find they don't care if they regain their desire. But if you are in a committed relationship with a man, he will care that you don't seem to want him. He will be 100 percent certain that if you don't want to have much sex with him, it means you don't love him anymore. He will be 100 percent certain that your lack of desire means you are having sex with someone else. Because this is his hormonal brain reality. If he loves you, he wants to have sex with you. If he doesn't want to have sex with you, he's probably getting it somewhere else, unless there is a health issue that is preventing erection. But no matter what you tell him about your hormones, he won't believe that the lights are off because the power is out. As I speak with more women in the Upgrade, they tell me that this very difference in hormonal state of mind has been a source of tremendous stress and sadness in their relationship.

With the exception of the hormonal storm of new love, male and female sex drives are almost always unmatched. Just as ours tanks, though, he might be taking Viagra or testosterone, making the gap even wider. My patient Michelle is a sixty-three-year-old teacher still working full time. Her husband, sixty-nine, is still running his packaging and shipping business. He is taking testosterone, and there is a brewing resentment about how his needs shape her life. "If I don't organize my day so that we have sex every morning, our relationship becomes a living hell," she said. "He's awful to be around. Once I get into it, it's okay, and it's nice to have an orgasm, but I don't crave it as much anymore. I'd rather just get out of bed in the morning and get on with my day."

For many women in the Upgrade, a vibrator does just fine for having an orgasm. "You lose the need to have a face in front of you when you have an orgasm," said Doris, eighty-one. "And the desire for one also becomes less urgent." Another woman, when asked if she minded if her husband slept with other women, said, "Not anymore. It's one less time I have to have sex."

The dynamic of the conversation about the gap can be dehumanizing for both partners. He can feel as though we are reducing him to a brutish animal, derided for having a drive that we no longer have. And his insistence on needing to *put it in* can make us feel like a blowup doll.

There is no place for women to talk about the standoff going on in so many homes. "I developed a repertoire of excuses," says Janet. "It's too late, and you know I have so much trouble sleeping. . . . I'll have to get up and wash because I keep getting bladder infections, and I'm just too tired. . . . I don't feel good about my body. . . . I'm exhausted. . . . I have a headache. . . . My back/hip/knee/neck hurts. Sergio started snapping back sarcastically with things like 'Oh, wait, there is a speck of dust on the floorboards. I have to clean it, so I can't have sex.'"

We need permission to open the dialogue so that we can understand each other. Without sex, he will feel crabby, unwanted, panicky, and unloved, just as we do when he shuts down and shuts us out. That same feeling of destabilization and fear that the relationship is ending when he won't talk is exactly what he feels when we don't want to have sex. It's how his brain is wired. And by fifty-five, his testosterone has been dropping for fifteen years, and the lower level drags his confidence down with it. He'll be looking for more reassurance from you because of it, and that emotional reassurance comes from the physical intimacy of making love.

"Sergio and I learned to talk about his need as an emotional yearning for connection," said Janet. "We were able to see that we suffered similarly through lack of intimacy of different kinds. When he shuts down and won't talk, I feel panicked about whether or not he loves me. I finally got it that when we don't make love, he feels panicked about whether or not I love him. So when he asks for connection, for feeling loved again, for feeling at peace, then I can respond to that." Since our sex drive isn't motivated by hormones anymore, it has to be activated by other means. Emotion and connection can do it for women. The men in the second half who learn this will get laid more often by using language she can hear. "I need sex [for my health or for my prostate]" will get the door slammed in men's faces.

Talking, connection through intimate conversation, is what sparks joy in the female brain, even during the Upgrade. Janet started calling it "girl sex." "Sergio and I had to learn to balance both girl sex and boy sex, and that means we've had to make sure we have quality time together every day," she continued. "If we each get our different needs for connection met, things are good between us. If we lose one aspect, we both get crabby."

Before the quiet of the Upgrade, the storm of hormone spikes in the Transition can kick up libido in wild bursts. For Beth, forty-seven was a crazy year. "I split with my husband, and I was like a teenager. I found my inner Samantha. She took over and I couldn't get enough. I got into bed with my boyfriend on a Sunday afternoon, and by the time I looked at the clock again, six hours had gone by." She was experiencing a double hit of hormones: Transition waves and the novelty that comes with a new partner. "It was short-lived," she said with some sadness in her voice. "By the time heavy bleeding started, I could feel the drive draining out of me. After the Transition was over, so was my libido."

Regardless of phase, Transition or Upgrade, and regardless of age, hormones can still kick up in your seventies and eighties with new love. "I'm not going to stick with the schlub I'm seeing," said Jean, "but for now, we are going at it like teenagers." Another patient of mine, a widow at seventy-two, was dating the husband of her late best friend. After a few months she broke it off, saying, "I'm just not that sexually attracted to him. It wouldn't be fair to continue, because I want him to have that joy in his life. I'm just not that into him sexually. I'm not into mercy screws." She wanted chemistry and wanted that for him too.

I opted not to keep taking testosterone when mine dropped. I tried it and didn't like how irritable it made me feel. It felt counter to the Upgrade in how it pushed the brain to hold on to the striving of the fertility phase. Just think what it would be like if, in the second half, you had the sex drive of a nineteen-year-old. How would it change the priorities of each day? We'd think more about sexy clothes, makeup, and seeking male attention, all the things we did to find partners during the fertility phase. I realized that wasn't how I wanted to live in my sixties and beyond. It was one thing to be consumed by these drives when I had my whole life ahead of me. It's another when I can count the average remaining years in front of me on my fingers and toes. I can remember my mother saying to me and my friend Janet over lunch when I was in my forties and she was in her midsixties, "Girls, frankly, I'm not so interested anymore, and I've had enough good sex to last me the rest of my life." In the Upgrade we have the chance to escape the control of hormone-driven thought and behavior. Like everything else, it's a personal decision, different for everyone.

Stage 3: Nothing Left to Lose

"My granddaughter turned to me one day," said Sylvia, "and asked the most surprising question. She wanted to know if my proximity to death was changing the way I thought about living."

"And what did you say?" I wondered how she'd address this concern of an eleven-year-old.

"I told her of course it changes everything," Sylvia responded. "How could it not?"

She saw the surprise on my face. "I had to be straight with her," Sylvia continued. "The big lesson for me was watching Robert die of cancer. He was so frightened, so completely freaked out. I had tried to talk to him about dying for many years, but he just kept slamming the door on the conversation. It was torture seeing him go through it with so much distress. But it's understandable. We don't talk about it in our culture. We don't examine it. We spend our lives pretending it won't happen. And I didn't want my granddaughter to grow up feeling the same way."

Facing change, loss, and death is another developmental phase that is not mapped, whether it occurs in the second half or, tragically out of time and place, early in life. Grief over dramatic change, including the loss of our own lives, is inevitable. Psychology doesn't treat any of this as a developmental stage but as episodic, as though it were optional, something surprising that might or might not happen across what is assumed to be the ideal of a steady flow of growth. Change and loss are seen as hiccups instead of what they really are: the actual condition of life itself. Change and loss happen with every heartbeat and breath, and without them, there would be no life, no nervous system and brain to power us. Without change and loss, the generation of neurochemical processes that influence our feelings, thoughts and actions, body and mind, would be dead, static, frozen. The opposite of alive. The opposite of engaged.

Change and loss manifest in every stage of life, and in the second half of life, all the discomforts of disease, illness, aging, and limitations are on steroids. Lost roles, lost partners, lost children, lost communities, lost friends, and confrontation with the reality of losing your own life. All of it can feel like an endless series of tornadoes crashing through our emotional lives. Relationships, homes, and the cities we live in change. The older we get, the more dramatic change we experience, in ourselves and our loved ones. "I lost eight people in one year," Natalie told me, reacting as though this were inconceivable. It's not. It's normal. It's life; it's death.

But to the nervous system, dramatic change is inconceivable. The nervous system craves certainty and stability in order to do the one job it has: keeping us alive. Yet the craving of the nervous system is in direct opposition to reality, and that is a major source of suffering. The more we accommodate the nervous system's delusion, the harder it is to manage the inevitable when it arrives, the harder it is to allow the tent of "Me" to adjust to rapidly shifting circumstances. Psychology may point out this issue, but it doesn't provide effective tools for shifting our experience of permanence to match the reality of impermanence.

There is no sugarcoating that life ends in death. Since the job of the brain and nervous system is survival, there will be nothing viscerally comfortable in this statement or in its exploration. Just the mention fires up the adrenals, squeezing out a massive flood of threat hormones, turning the survival instinct on full blast in the brain. The natural response is to try to close the door on the source of discomfort. But turning away can spiral us out into a debilitating death anxiety. When fear goes underground, it has a nasty tendency to be transformed into chronic stress. Persistent denial shuts off our problem-solving capacity. Instead of recruiting our creativity for addressing reality, our ingeniousness ends up scaffolding more delusion, like *I will not die, somehow*. Distress builds and reality breaks through, no matter how hard we try to block it out.

I get it. It's hard to face death. We would rather live in denial and take the consequences. But to complete the Upgrade, there is a quality-of-life and quality-of-death decision to be made. There is growth and opportunity right up until the very end. But first we have to look the fear right in the face. If you're already experiencing some strong feelings and need to take a break, go ahead. If you're ready to ask the hard questions, let's go.

Stage 4: Facing the Monster Under the Bed

Terri remembered asking her mother at age three if everybody dies. "My mother said yes. Then I asked her if I was going to die. She responded, 'Yes, but not for a very long time, so don't worry about it.'" What that fairly typical conversation does is teach avoidance as coping: Just don't think about it. "And I remember," Terri said, "that I became much more anxious even in that moment. That fear resurfaced as full-blown anxiety when I faced big health issues in my twenties."

After a lifetime of the worry echoing in our brain circuits, death anxiety can take control of our lives, wrecking the time we have left by keeping us from being present to what's right in front of us as fear becomes a filter for everything. It's not fun for us, and it's not a picnic for those who end up being our fear's punching bags. The only way to deal with that anxiety is to open the door and face it.

"My friend Rosa had breast cancer that had metastasized to the bone, and she fought dying with all her might," said Terri. "She was miserable. She was in constant pain from useless procedures she demanded in the vain hope of prolonging her life. She screamed at everyone, alienating caretakers, friends, and family. It was awful to witness. Even at the end, she wouldn't let anyone use the word 'cancer' in her presence. She died terrified, clutching at the bed." If we don't look death in the face, the stress and threat systems remain in low-grade, chronic activation. Attuning to reality is part of how humans heal, especially when we can't be cured.

"I was in my early twenties and I was single in New York, just out of the hospital from a second major surgery, when the AIDS crisis was in full bloom," said Terri. "We lived in a constant state of terror. It was before we really knew how it was transmitted, and we were all afraid we'd picked it up somehow."

I remember those days in San Francisco. So many young people were suffering and dying. For those of us who stood on the sidelines, our personal fear collided with a global health crisis. For some it can be a recipe for collapse. But Terri chose another way.

"I decided to run headlong in the direction of my fear," she said. "I read everything I could. I learned about the newly emerging hospice movement. I sat at bedsides and held hands with friends I was losing. I did everything I could to be present for them as fearlessly as possible. I started to understand a bit more about the process, seeing how sensitive their nervous systems became, how much peace and solitude they needed. So I ran interference with difficult family members and made sure rowdy friends who might trigger painful memories had short visits. I left false optimism, false hope, and the imposition of my own grief at the door. It's the last thing a dying person needs. It might make us feel good, but it stresses them out."

The psychological intervention cognitive behavioral therapy (CBT) is particularly effective in addressing anxiety and full-blown phobias. One of the tactics is called exposure therapy. In her twenties Terri, like many of us, hadn't experienced the loss of many people in her life. To address her fear, she instinctively sought out the experience in her own form of exposure therapy. Familiarity gave her the courage to begin to open the door to her own mortality.

When I got sick in London during medical school and no one knew what was wrong with me, I was so depleted I felt I might die. But being gravely ill at a developmental stage when your peers are getting revved up for life can be isolating. It was for me, and it was for Terri.

The courage to face death anxiety is different in the Upgrade. We have a database of experience: loss of friends and family, our own brush with death, or a frightening series of tests. We've spent years wondering what's going to take us out, and at this stage we know it's going to be something sooner or later. We've participated in plenty of frightening dress rehearsals. In the aftermath, the adrenals power down, the parasympathetic nervous system turns on, we relax, we breathe, we smile, and we sleep . . . until reality sets in once again. It may feel counterintuitive to walk right into the heart of anxiety when everything in your brain and nervous system may tell you that facing death will bring it on faster. But just as with the monster under the bed, we have to look at it in order to quell our fear.

I was thinking back to a friend's grandmother, who didn't have any spiritual beliefs but read Sherwin Nuland's bestseller *How We Die* and said it gave her peace. Nuland, a physician who was also my professor at

Yale, wrote of the various ways the body shuts down as it approaches death. Knowing what could take place physically helped my friend's grandmother attune to what was actually happening instead of clinging to what she wished were happening. Her internal adjustment sparked a shift from the crankiness of loss to the joy of the present. Her family noticed the difference in her personality. She was more fun than ever to be around. She wrote out her medical directives and had her DNR (do not resuscitate) order taped to the wall above her bed, so that if a caregiver called an ambulance, she'd have a better chance of having her wishes respected. When she realized she was near death, and her son needed to go abroad for work, she told him to go. "I might not be here when you get back," she said, "but I'll see you another time."

Stage 5: Facing the Dying Brain and Body

When my mother was dying, my brother was told to take her home so that she could be in familiar surroundings and receive hospice care. For days all four siblings talked with her, held her hand, stroked her head, and tried to make her feel loved. My sister and I helped her into the bathroom one morning so that she could have a bowel movement. We brought her back to bed, and after some time the hospice nurse had us leave the room. Shortly after we complied, our mother passed. In our desire to comfort her and make her feel loved, our touch had caused too much peripheral stimulation, which had to be quieted in order for her to leave. Many years of practice and lots of anecdotal evidence make it clear that people need solitude and they need their loved ones to give them space to focus on their own process. It's hard for loved ones of the gregarious. It's a reversal that may feel like a rejection, but their need for you not to be there is a reflection of how deep their attachment is.

I watched how my mother changed, how totally peaceful and loving she became, how open and accepting of everyone she came into contact with. The kind of emotional and spiritual growth she went through made it clear that facing death is a developmental stage. If we don't align with the reality of it, we miss a huge opportunity to enlarge our playing field as wisdom fills our tent of "Me." We can be very brave and compassionate when we are fully, joyfully, tragically present.

When we don't understand the developmental stage, we will say and do the wrong things for others at every turn. "My friend Rosa," said Terri, "when she was dying of breast cancer, limited visitors to just a few of us. It was too hard for her to be around those who were out of tune with her process, who couldn't be present to it." Feelings were hurt because of lack of understanding.

The outer signs of dying—the sunken cheeks, eyes, and temples, the translucent pallor of the skin, the glassy eyes and lack of focus—are not hard to spot. Having to pee a lot, a feeling of heaviness in the limbs, inability to swallow easily, are all signs that the body is shutting down. The nervous system becomes very sensitive to others' moods and energy, harsh sounds, bright lights. The late stages bring a slowing of the breath, some difficulty breathing, and the need for lots of sleep. There can be a last-minute surge of energy and clarity—many report long, deep, meaningful conversations hours before a loved one departs.

Researchers are beginning to collect stories of the less tangible indicators of the proximity of death. Buffalo, New York, hospice physician Christopher Kerr has compiled more than a thousand cases for a peer-reviewed study indicating the commonality of experiences at the end of life. Of particular interest to him has been waking, conscious experiences of interactions with loved ones who have already passed. These experiences are real to those who have them, and they occur while wide awake. He learned during his experience with the AIDS crisis that no matter how a patient seemed to be doing physically, as soon as they had one of these experiences, it meant that death was near, almost always within days or weeks.

As doctors and researchers collect more information and first-person accounts of the dying, new questions are being asked about the relationship between the brain and consciousness. For more than a century, medicine has labeled consciousness as an epiphenomenon of the brain, meaning it is assumed that consciousness arises out of the brain, but there is no explanation for why this happens. The other assumption is that the brain must be in a state of neurochemical and structural organization and awake for consciousness to function. But the advent of resuscitation medicine in the 1970s has begun to shift the thinking.

Near-death experiences (NDEs) have been recorded across time and culture, but the number of people having them grew exponentially in the last third of the twentieth century. More and more people were emerging from surgery or resuscitation with detailed knowledge of conversations and instruments used, as well as reports of spiritual experiences that were practically the same. In fact, one British researcher, Sam Parnia, who is a professor at New York University's Langone Medical Center, worked closely with ICU doctors in New York to study the connection between consciousness and wakefulness. They came into rooms in which patients were not awake and hung paintings for a period of time. They removed the paintings before the patients awoke, and a surprising percentage asked their caregivers what had happened to the paintings. Consciousness was working without wakefulness, and Parnia will be setting up more studies to confirm the findings.

In death, the heart stops but the brain doesn't at first. Connections between synapses happen through electricity generated by neurochemicals. Brain cells suck up the last of the blood's oxygen and hang on as long as they can. There is a surge of serotonin, which may be responsible for a tremendous feeling of peace reported by many. When the oxygen runs out, a tsunami of reactions halt the neurochemical electricity in the cells. The lights, so to speak, are turned off pretty much all at once.

It was always assumed that when the brain becomes disorganized in this process, consciousness shouldn't be able to function. But it does in NDEs. Neuroscience is proving that you can be awake and not be conscious. No one is saying that people have died and come back, but we are able to confirm that consciousness is occurring at a moment when not only is wakefulness impossible but life itself might not be possible. And in those experiences, people commonly report exquisite clarity, expansive and immersive feelings of love and compassion, and a visceral sense of the continuation and vastness of consciousness itself.

Maybe it's strange that a neuroscientist is talking about these experiences. It feels a bit odd for me to be exploring how the brain and biology are intertwined with spiritual experience. For someone who has spent most of my life finding a material cause for feeling states, this is new. It is the brain and nervous system that mediate our experience of reality, our visceral sense of what is real, right, and true, so it makes sense that there might be spiritual answers too in neurochemistry and neurobiology. The question of consciousness and the brain has opened a whole new field of contemplative neuroscience and exploration into why NDEs and even the use of psilocybin (the psychotropic chemical in psychedelic mushrooms) can wipe away the fear of death for many.

I haven't made up my mind about a lot of it, but as a scientist I think it's important to remain open to mystery.

Stage 6: Planning for a Good Death

Developmentally we spend our late childhood through early adult years expanding and practicing the use of the prefrontal cortex (PFC) to solve, plan, decide, anticipate risks and rewards, all in the process of solving the puzzle of what makes up a good life. We do it so that we get our priorities straight and so that our days and relationships are full of quality. Our health is absolutely part of the equation, but improving our health span adds only about two and a half years to our life span. I think it's equally important to quality of life to ask what makes a good death, to calm the fear circuits and begin to recruit the PFC to the task.

If family and friends were to say to each other, "She had a good death," what would that mean? In my family, it meant that all of the siblings were able to be peaceful around our mother, to show our love for one another during the last two weeks of her life. My mother told us what she wanted, and we worked on her memorial together, her at the kitchen table, me on the floor, patting her knees. She said she couldn't believe we were planning her final transition together, and she made it clear she didn't want anyone to wear black or to mourn. She wanted a joyful, loving, God-filled celebration of her life, so I went out and bought a hot-pink minidress with rhinestones. My sister wore a bright woven jacket my mother had brought back from Guatemala. No one behaved badly, and that had a lot to do with the tone of unconditional love set by my mother. It allowed all of us to share a space of reverence, respect, and dignity, to be present enough to feel the enormity of her passing.

We can each harness the power of daydreaming, imagination, and innovation that we have used to build a good life and visualize a snapshot of the deathbed scene we want, the feelings we want our loved ones to come away with. What would that look and feel like for us?

Maybe we can begin with what we don't want it to feel like, the burdens we might have been left with that we'd like not to place on our loved ones because of unfinished business. Birth and death, our two big transitions, often happen in an overly medicalized hospital setting. Maybe that's what we want, to fight medically until the last. Or maybe being surrounded by strangers; bright lights; whirring, beeping machines; constant procedures; and separation from loved ones might cause too much distress. There is no such thing as a perfect death. But what makes a good death for you needs to be defined and talked about. It's as important as a good life.

There are so many practice opportunities if we stop to think. A mammogram, waiting for clarifying results of an abnormal test, even a checkup can be a source of much more anxiety at this stage. We've been through it with others, holding their hands, seeing the different outcomes. To be clear: not the same as going through it yourself. Those were dress rehearsals. Your own is not. Facing it down yourself is another matter.

There are lots of resources on how to manage the phase when the doctors give up on you, to grieve the loss of your own life, and to map out palliative care. But how the visceral brain-and-nervous system aspect is influenced by emotion and thoughts is important to respect. I know I want to find my way to calm, peace, and clarity. In his book *Good Life, Good Death*, Tibetan lama Gehlek Rimpoche wrote that a good death begins with a good life, one of practicing "patience, love, and compassion in your daily life." And regardless of our habit, he strongly recommends we plan and think about it well ahead of time, because when we are actually dying, it will be too late to say what we need to say or to create the circumstances for the transition we want to have. There are communities, death cafés, death doulas, and more who can shed light on the process, guides who can help us learn to focus on creating the most supportive internal and external environments. By connecting with the helpers who can address the terrors in the night, we are triggering calming neurochemicals of bonding; mirror neurons come into play as we begin to match the emotional state of an experienced guide. The brain and nervous system can support the Upgrade right up until the very end. Working with this is a rest-of-your-life process.

I WILL UPGRADE!

Chapter 16

*Women are born with pain built in. It's our physical destiny—period pains,
sore boobs, childbirth. We carry it within ourselves throughout our
lives. . . . We have pain on a cycle for years and years and years, and then
just when you feel you are making peace with it all, what happens? The
menopause comes. The fucking menopause comes and it is the most
wonderful fucking thing in the world. Yes, your entire pelvic floor crumbles
and you get fucking hot and no one cares, but then you're free. . . . You're
just a person.*

—Belinda, Fleabag, *season 1*

There is a reason this soliloquy has been repeated and shared relentlessly
since the moment it aired: It's true. For me, hearing it was a turning point
in getting this book finished. The Upgrade is an exquisite portal into the
best years of our lives. I wrote it to start, not end, the conversation about
it, and I hope we will all contribute to creating a new map of the second
half together.

I've learned through my journey that the Upgrade is not about reaching some mythical plane of awareness. It's a deeper engagement with and

understanding of this life, this world, this body, this mind. It's remembering to listen to the part of myself that knows the truth of who I am and how things work, the truth of my relationships, successes, and failures, all that I deafened my ears to during the reproductive years in order to keep the peace, the status quo. Blocking out the truth made me at times feel like I was about to lose my mind, and I never understood why that feeling dogged me. But with the earplugs of the fertile phase removed, I can learn to hear what my own will is asking for again, lifting the lid of internal strife created by the competing priorities of what my biology was dictating and who I am as a woman.

The pacemaker of your nervous system and brain changes in the Upgrade, providing a beat that supports emerging out of who we thought we were in the fertile phase into who we actually are. I find I have become deeply interested in improving the tent of "Me," facing, accepting, and adjusting faults; finding ways to bring out the best I have to give, in order to be effective in offering it up every day.

For me, human potential, personal growth, has become real in the Upgrade. I finally have the willingness to see how some of my old emotional and behavioral patterns bring suffering to others and to myself; that realization is compelling me to find effective ways to change. In wanting to be the best version of myself, I seek out a reliable plan, a program with clear goals, clear results, and support from others who have succeeded in doing what I am attempting to do.

There are people to learn from in a way that is different from how we have learned in the past. I find I have to be willing to be shaken to my core, to have a fearless look at my own tent, at what doesn't serve anymore, to weed out the parts of my character that are harmful and consciously fertilize the good parts, helping them grow. The result is more peace, more joy. I have earned the right to pursue this in the Upgrade.

I most often see patients for the first time during a crisis in their thirties or forties, and almost always a huge part of solving their issue is around hormones and/or antidepressants. When they are stable enough, they leave therapy. Often, some fifteen years later they will circle back, having been brought to their knees again by life's events. They are past the fertile phase of hormonal waves, and so I no longer start with medications or hormones for most. I listen carefully to hear what remains broken from the past. I also look for where they have already stepped onto the path of the Upgrade and find ways to turn their attention to that path in order to continue. I want to know what they are doing to care for themselves. We consider meditative and spiritual resources to help them fertilize the best in them and to weed out what's choking their garden. I do my best to help them disable the hamster wheel of worry. I begin showing them how to wire feelings of safety and self-compassion through meditative techniques instead of looking to medication to temporarily create those pathways. By using cognitive practices, they more easily find the strength to fix the broken parts and to continue the Upgrade.

Scientists have now shown that it's possible to dial up or down just about any cognitive or behavioral trait—aggression, compulsion, sociability, learning, memory, compassion, gratitude—in the brain's soft wiring by means of various interventions, whether chemical or meditative. Prozac can make the shy bold and the solemn cheerful. Compassion meditation can melt the fearful into courageous openheartedness. If some may see this as manipulative of our own genetic or epigenetic destiny, well, so be it. The tent of "Me" is more under our control than most of us realize. And I celebrate this widening of possibility.

There is no road map for making changes to our nervous system and brain; I'm building my own and sharing it with you to encourage you to build your own as you go. What are the qualities we value, and what neural support would we like to give ourselves? This brain is *OUR* brain, this story is *OUR* story; it's up to us to ask ourselves who we want to be in the Upgrade and to learn what is possible to achieve.

Like dieting, attending to shifting what's in the tent of "Me" requires sticking to a plan and accepting that change doesn't happen overnight. But if we spend as much time on the Upgrade as we did on weight control and appearance in the fertility phase, our tent of "Me" will be awesome.

Upgrading takes courage, but without it we walk backward into old age, obsessed with the past. Going down memory lane, reminiscing in retirement, is an old model in which we abandon growth and shrink into senility. I want to walk wholeheartedly into the future, with my eyes on the way ahead.

Fear kills microglia, the cells in the brain we need to keep it nourished and clean. When remodeling the tent of "Me," it's important to consider the impact of fear and look for the helpers who can support us in unearthing the courage we need. There will be people who won't want you to remodel your tent. They will fight you. You may have to move them out of the inner circle, away from the tent pole. What I've found is that those who support us in the way we need often show up rather magically.

Pregnant with Compassion

When the huge responsibility for family and little kids is unplugged, it unleashes decision-making bandwidth as never before. When the near ones don't factor so heavily into daily life choices, the love brain has a chance to expand. The neurocircuitry of the love brain and tent of "Me" can now enlarge. What's included will feel new, weird, and maybe even selfish: What's best for "Me" takes priority in a new way; and the impulse to act on what's best for others outside the family can fill us with a new motivation to act.

The spirit of altruism seeps into the second half, sometimes for the first time. You see suffering outside the family and want to help. The grandmothering impulse, the nurturing maternal instinct, may creep in even for women who haven't had their own children. I've seen it drive women in the Upgrade on a mission to become a peer role model, to share what we've learned with other women in this phase of life. It's a key imperative, to walk this road with enough people so that it is no longer a semisecret trail in the woods but a superhighway with very clear signage. In order to be ready to embrace this role, we have to think about our health. We give primacy to longevity and health because we have work to do. We are needed to mother the world.

The first part of life was primarily about becoming self-conscious, and wanting to come out ahead in comparison to others. The Upgrade is about unwinding self-consciousness into a generosity toward ourselves and others, shifting the focus to becoming who we wished we'd met when we were younger. Becoming, for others, the person we needed to help us through life.

In the optimized Upgrade, women fight for women. We get daughters out of bad marriages; we help our granddaughters rebel, our nieces succeed. I know with my nieces I am often a sounding board, once in a while the source of some much-needed extra cash in an emergency, and a neutral shoulder to cry on in the wake of some bad decisions. Being real rather than nice becomes a gift to others.

In the Upgrade we learn to refuse to accept unacceptable behavior from others—and from ourselves. The old rhythms of the fertility phase, the traces of those habits, will always remain, ready to be pricked in the circuits of my heart, gut, and brain. So I am vigilant to make sure I counterbalance those pulls by enhancing the circuits of the Upgrade. I've learned to meet my own needs more and stop expecting that they be met by others. I've worked on building the confidence to tell the truth and being willing to pay the price for speaking my truth. I've learned to tell my story without flinching, and I've become a boundary-setting ninja. I've learned to say what I mean and mean what I say, and try my best to do it without saying it mean. It's better for me and it's better for everyone around me.

Reaching out to the younger generation becomes an imperative. I think of Elizabeth Warren's tireless selfies and pinky promises with little girls as she asked them during her 2020 presidential campaign to step into power when they grow up.

Becoming the Woman We Needed to See

The Talmud states, "Do not be daunted by the enormity of the world's grief. Do justly now, love mercy now, walk humbly now. You are not obligated to complete the work, but neither are you free to abandon it."

So often I've felt in the Upgrade that we come into a full appreciation of being female just as society writes us off. But there is a vast historical library of female vocal authority in Eleanor Roosevelt, Shirley Chisholm,

Dolores Huerta, Carol Moseley Braun, Ann Richards, Toni Morrison, Jane Goodall, Maya Angelou, Angela Merkel, Ruth Bader Ginsburg, Sonia Sotomayor, Marie Yovanovitch, Fiona Hill, Stacey Abrams, Greta Thunberg, and Kamala Harris, America's first female vice president. Even *we* forget when we hear those voices.

It's not easy to step into our power. When we don't introject secondary status as expected, we are brutalized from all sides. If you don't believe me, name one woman who stepped out of her gender role who hasn't been attacked outrageously. What's different in the Upgrade is how much less the familiar onslaught gets under our skin.

With the quieting of the ovaries' caretaking hormones we have the opportunity not to let any of it cut us deeply, as it did during the fertile phase, when oxytocin would spark an apocalyptic fire in the nervous system, telling us the world was coming to an end if one single person disliked us. In the Upgrade, we can speak our minds, knowing we will not be destroyed by the fire we draw.

In another era we would have been called a battle ax. Now we are badasses. We are becoming leaders in the Upgrade. What do some of our most formidable, fearless leaders have in common? They're women who came to the fullness of their powers on the other side of menopause, and now they're running Congress (Nancy Pelosi), running for president (Elizabeth Warren, Kamala Harris, Amy Klobuchar), sitting on the Supreme Court (RBG, rest in power, Sonia Sotomayor, Elena Kagan). Think of Christine Lagarde, Patti Smith, Ruth E. Carter, Sister Helen Prejean— all forces to be reckoned with as younger women, but none of them as deeply visionary, as thoroughly glorious, as when they got to the other side.

No longer the crazy old crone in the attic, we are emerging into a world in which we are taking more control than ever.

I WILL UPGRADE

I'm tired of having yet another bar to rise to, I found myself thinking about the Upgrade. But what I've learned is that seeing that I'm worth more than I ever imagined allows the Upgrade to flow naturally. I just need to get out of the way of its unfolding. I want to give myself the best chance for a bright future, and I hope you give yourself and the women around you that chance too.

Like everyone, I drag my previous selves behind me. Although I occasionally look back, I try not to stare. I've learned to love myself in my own eyes, not in everyone else's. I feel gratitude for having this once-in-a-lifetime opportunity to make the transition into the Upgrade.

My friend Janet went through many crises in her early years: disastrous relationships, dire illness, dislocation of work taking her to a country she never wanted to live in. In the Upgrade she sat alone in a restaurant in Paris having a last indulgent meal before heading into a retreat. "And I told my younger self," she recalled, "who was so freaked out by all the change, not to worry, that everything would be just fine. It's not that my outer circumstances had changed. It's that inside I was at peace with whatever happened."

Age wrinkles your skin; loss of enthusiasm wrinkles the soul. I will not let my being shrivel. I hope you won't let yours either. I was never entirely ready for anything in my life, and I'm not always ready for the Upgrade either. But to get myself psyched up, I thrust my arms up to the sky and shout, often, to no one and everyone, "I WILL UPGRADE!" It helps trigger the brain and nervous system to generate enthusiasm for becoming who I want to be: less jealous, more open, a warmer heart, a wiser mind.

Visualize your future, your Upgrade. Start by thinking about how you want to feel and who you want to be an hour from now. Work your way up to a day, a week, a month, a year. Visualize and fake it till you make it. It will materialize if you can see it. It will materialize if you remain willing to engage in solving the puzzle of your life until the very end. I look forward to meeting you in the Upgrade.

Appendix

I wanted to create a few shortcuts so that you'd easily be able to find the actionables that emerge from the book. I hope this might help you create your own plan for optimizing your cognitive and emotional superpowers in the Upgrade.

Daily: Before getting out of bed, I wiggle my toes and smile, practice EFTs, essential first thoughts: say good morning to God, meditate, and pray that I might be of use to others by being kind, easygoing, and calm. I ask for the courage to be direct, honest, and patient; and to keep my mouth shut when I shouldn't speak, especially when people need to learn things on their own without my interference. I stretch, squeeze my butt cheeks (to strengthen glutes), and get bright morning light for fifteen to twenty minutes (in winter I use a full spectrum lamp); I do moderate exercise in pool aerobics, reclining bike, dance on my deck, and eat a Mediterranean diet with fifteen hours of intermittent fasting (no food after 6:00 P.M.). I supplement with vitamin D_3, magnesium, CoQ10, vitamin K, and a fiber supplement. I take my medications: rosuvastatin (a statin drug), levothyroxine (thyroid hormone), and an estradiol patch. I aim to go to sleep at 10:30 P.M. and wake at 7:00 A.M.

Upgrade Principles to Honor

- Circadian rhythms: Sleep is key to cognition and control of inflammation. If you can manage to make a habit of getting to bed by 11:00 P.M. at the latest—in bed with screens off at ten thirty—you will set yourself up for success the following day. You'll be more alert and more energetic, and you'll want to engage in the movement your brain needs to power cognition.
- Waking up one hour earlier than usual, and sleeping earlier, gives you a double-digit improvement in mood and protection from depression.
- Move to stay alive: It will improve your mood, preserve cognition, battle melancholy, reduce inflammation, and remind your brain and body that you still need them to keep pumping because you've got a lot left to do in the world. If you can't take HT, movement, even if it's just your arms, is your cognitive safety net.
- Eat for the Upgrade by defeating inflammation and feeding your muscles: Limit carbs, grains, and fruits; lower animal fat as much as possible; rely mainly on protein, healthy fats, and veggies for optimal functioning.
- Stimulate your memory by staying engaged and by exercising. Squeeze your glutes 100 times a day. Engaging and strengthening this key core muscle for standing, balancing, and walking will help you reap maximum cerebellum benefits.
- I believe in snacks! Movement and meditation snacks, that is. Don't make change insurmountable by thinking you have to run a marathon or start a monthlong silent retreat tomorrow. Start with "snacks." Movement snacks of ten minutes—stretching, a quick walk, some quick work with weights—can be the foundation for building a new habit. The same goes for meditation: If you haven't done it before or very much, the mind's attention muscles won't be strong, so expecting to remain calm and focused for more than a minute or two is unrealistic. Even the Dalai Lama recommends

starting with thirty seconds a few times a day. A friend of mind uses the Breathe app on her Apple Watch for daily reminders.

- Calm the nervous system: It's going to be key to clearheaded decision making. Sleep and exercise are huge; so are breathing and meditation. Recommendations for practices are in "Supportive Modalities for the Upgrade" below.

Set Yourself Up for Sleep

- Go to bed at the same time every night.
- Get at least fifteen minutes of bright morning light every sunny day, forty minutes on cloudy days (use a full spectrum light lamp in winter).
- Do something physical that makes you a little tired before 2:00 P.M., cardio and strength. You need to stay active so that your brain registers that your nerves and muscles are still in strong need of its services. Otherwise both your brain and muscles start to weaken. There's a strong correlation between leg strength and mental acuity over age eighty: The stronger your legs, the sharper your mind.
- Focus on eating as many nonstarchy vegetables as you can manage in a day, and have lean protein with every meal; consume under 100 grams of carbs per day. You can use a carb counting app to track. Learn to eat to best feed the body, and see if you can't take a hard look at emotional eating—I know when I reach for ice cream and peanut butter, I'm not actually hungry, so I try to distract myself to keep from setting off harmful inflammation. If you keep the body happy and healthy, you don't want to wreck it.
- Eat eggs, turkey, or cottage cheese a couple of times per week; choline from egg yolks helps with sleep and memory, as does tryptophan in turkey and cottage cheese.
- Consume omega-3 fatty acids that cross the blood-brain barrier. I eat salmon several times a week because most omega supplements

don't cross the blood-brain barrier as well as food does. You can get omegas in chia and flaxseeds too.

- Minimize caffeine. My one cup of coffee in the morning is two-thirds decaf, one-third caffeinated, and that's it for the day, unless I'm determined not to sleep!
- Alcohol doesn't suit. It causes hot flashes, makes your hands red and swollen, and makes you sleepy at the wrong time. Two hours after your last drink the brain becomes alert. Mostly, you'll fall asleep quickly, then wake in the middle of the night and have a helluva time getting back to sleep. If you really want to drink, lunch on a weekend is best. To keep people from thinking I'm antisocial at dinners, I let the host pour, and I may take a sip or two. If pressed, I'll say something like, "I'll feel better if I don't."
- Do intermittent fasting five days a week: Finish dinner by six or seven, exercise in the morning on an empty stomach, and eat breakfast around ten or eleven.
- Sleep seven to eight hours per night.
- Sleep with an eye mask and custom earplugs, and keep the room between sixty-five and sixty-eight degrees. It helps prevent wakefulness from ambient light and sounds in the room, and a low temperature helps you sleep.

Apnea

Be on the lookout: If you are sleeping through the night but waking up exhausted, if someone tells you that you snore, if you fall asleep within minutes of sitting down during the day, if you have a hard time staying awake through meetings or movies, if inflammation markers and blood pressure are rising, and if you're carrying more weight than is healthy, consider getting a sleep study to see if you might have undiagnosed sleep apnea. It's an incredibly dangerous condition in 10 to 20 percent of women that can cause heart attacks, brain fog, and strokes and has been linked to diabetes and cancer. Don't take it lightly. If your doctor prescribes a CPAP, wear it. It can take time to find one that's comfortable. Don't give up.

SSRI: Use for Hot Flashes and Depression

Estrogen is the gold standard for treating hot flashes, but for those who cannot take it and have severe hot flashes, an SSRI or SNRI is worth trying and in some women can reduce hot flashes by as much as 65 percent. They can also help with sleep. The SSRIs identified in studies as helpful are paroxetine (Paxil or Brisdelle), paroxetine extended release (Paxil CR), citalopram (Celexa), and escitalopram (Lexapro). Venlafaxine (Effexor XR) was identified as a potential first-line SNRI. Paroxetine extended release was the most effective at doses of both 12.5 milligrams per day and 25 milligrams per day. Venlafaxine worked more quickly on symptom relief than the SSRIs did, but in study participants there were more side effects like nausea and constipation. Fluoxetine (Prozac) and sertraline (Zoloft) work too. SNRIs may increase blood pressure, so if you have an issue with blood pressure, use extreme caution. For depression without hot flashes, buproprion (Wellbutrin), psychotherapy, and CBT (cognitive behavioral therapy) are well established treatments. The NAMS (North American Menopause Society) recommendations include the following SSRIs and SNRIs: paroxetine salt (Brisdelle) 7.5 milligrams per day; paroxetine or paroxetine extended release 10–25 milligrams per day; escitalopram 10–20 milligrams per day; citalopram 10–20 milligrams per day; desvenlafaxine 50–150 milligrams per day; and venlafaxine (Effexor XR) 37.5–150 milligrams per day. I agree with their recommendation to start at the lowest available dose and raise it in tiny increments if needed. I like working with the SSRIs you can get in liquid form, which allows me to individualize the dose more easily. All of them now come in liquid except Brisdelle, which comes only in 7.5 milligram doses. It is the only non-estrogen drug that is FDA approved for hot flashes. If you do start an SSRI or SNRI, remember to keep a regular and detailed mood and side-effect log. Some people have had dangerous emotional reactions. If you find yourself having suicidal ideation, talk to someone immediately, and get back to your doctor for help getting off or changing the drug. Don't attempt to stop it on your own. If no one is around, call the National Suicide Prevention Lifeline 24-7: 800-273-8255.

Alternate-Nostril Breathing

Known as nine-round breathing in some Buddhist circles, maybe you've been guided through this at a yoga class as well. It's a pretty widespread technique used in contemplative traditions for getting the mind to settle before meditation, prayer, or even before needing to focus at work.

Round 1: Sit up straight but relaxed. If you can sit on a cushion or the edge of a chair without support, it's great, but if you need support, please use it. Start by using your right hand to block your right nostril. Breathe in as slowly and quietly as possible through the left nostril. At the top of the breath, use the right hand to block the left nostril, and breathe out through the right nostril as slowly and quietly as possible. Breathe in through the left and out through the right three times.

Round 2: Without taking a break (unless you feel dizzy, in which case, stop, of course), switch the process, using your left hand to cover your left nostril. Breathe in through the right nostril as slowly and quietly as possible. At the top of the breath, use the left hand to block the right nostril, and breathe out through the left nostril as slowly and quietly as possible. Breathe in through the right and out through the left three times.

Round 3: Again without taking a break unless you are straining or are dizzy, breathe in and out through both nostrils three times at the same slow and quiet pace.

You can add a visualization of breathing in good, healing energy and breathing out a dark, smoky cloud of what no longer serves. You can do the nine rounds once or repeat them three, seven, or even twenty-one times.

Nurturing Moment Meditation

The following is an excerpt, reprinted with permission, from "The Compassion Shift," part of a twenty-one-day compassion challenge hosted by the Compassion Center at Emory University. It's an introduction to the foundational practice of Cognitively Based Compassion Training (CBCT). You can learn more at compassion.emory.edu. You can also find a guide to brief daily meditations there.

> When we feel safe and cared for it opens the door to possibility. Connecting with a personal experience of receiving kindness calms the body and mind, helping us to extend care and kindness to others.

Description

Born to a fifteen-year-old addict partnered with an abusive drug dealer, LaTonya Goffney's childhood was full of violence and uncertainty until she was nine. She found refuge at school, under the care of teachers who recognized her brilliance. She flourished after moving in with her grandmother, and went on to get a degree in education. As a superintendent, Goffney has embraced the challenge of turning around some of the most troubled school systems in Texas. The care and safety she received allowed her to thrive and to extend care and safety to other children, many times over.

Adversity can knock us out of what psychologists call our Zone of Wellbeing. The Zone of Wellbeing is an optimal physical and psychological balance. When our biological threat systems are calmed, the release of neurochemicals makes us feel strong and at peace, able to weather life's ups and downs. The Zone of Wellbeing is where we experience resilience, the ability to bounce back from adversity. We might experience it after a good night's sleep, a relaxing vacation, praise from a colleague, the embrace of a loved one, a joyful welcome from a beloved pet, a peaceful moment by a river, lake, or sea, a calming walk in nature, or an inspiring spiritual setting.

Having ready access to feelings of safety and emotional warmth bolsters resilience—our ability to bounce back from upsets and challenges, large or small. When we are able to recall or imagine feelings of refuge, nurturance, peace, or freedom, and when we remind ourselves of the benefits of these feelings, we can begin to have some influence over reentering and remaining more reliably in our Zone of Wellbeing. Research has shown that when our nervous system is balanced, our health improves, along with our ability to remain calm and think clearly even in difficult times.

Awakening to the value of kindness, of being safe and cared for, we become ready to venture beyond ourselves. If we can abide for a moment in a sense of security, it gives us the foundation to imagine how wonderful it would be if others could also feel safe and secure. It can motivate us to commit more wholeheartedly to compassion.

Before we begin the meditation, **Connecting to a Moment of Nurturance,** let's engage in a three- to five-minute writing exercise. Take a moment to find something to write with. Choose, or imagine, a moment of feeling secure, comforted, or nurtured. Don't worry about the story that came before or after that instant. Just see if you can isolate in your mind a soothing moment sitting by a river, receiving kindness from a stranger, support from a friend. Maybe it's a time in the arms of a loved one, or a family member. If you are alive today, you had a moment like this, whether you remember or not. Someone took care of you. Someone fed and nurtured you. So imagine what that might have felt like to be held and protected, safe, and comforted. Or remember how you felt holding a small child, or a time you were able to offer welcome comfort to someone in distress. Perhaps it is like when you dance, holding your partner close. Perhaps it is the experience of unconditional love from a pet who welcomes you home with joy. If you grew up near the sea or a lake, think of the peace of floating on calm pristine waters. If that moment of safety and security comes from a spiritual source, evoke that presence or figure, the place of worship, or the community itself.

Once you have chosen your moment of nurturance, write down as many details as you can remember or imagine, especially the sights, smells, sensations, textures, the feeling of the presence of others if they are involved.

With these in mind, let's get ready to meditate.

Meditation

Please take a moment to find a comfortable posture and connect with your body and current feelings. If you notice tension in any part of the body, feel free to stretch or move gently to help relax. You may close your eyes or keep them slightly open. Feel your body in your seat, and allow yourself to settle into the present experience.

When ready, take a few deep breaths if it is comfortable to do so. Gently inhale, and if you like, have the sense that nourishing air, rich with oxygen, is infusing your entire being. As you breathe out, see if you can release tensions and worries to some degree to allow the body and mind to settle into an unfolding sense of calm or ease.

Let's now take a moment to bring to mind a nurturing moment: something that makes us feel better, safer, or happier. When have we experienced that? In nature? While being cared for—by a friend or loved one, or a mentor, or a figure from a faith tradition? If such a resource does not come to mind, see if we can just imagine a person, or an environment, that would support feeling safer or better.

Choosing one, let's take a moment to immerse ourselves in this experience by bringing it to mind as vividly as we can. Where is this scene happening? What do we see; which colors, textures; what's the light like? What about the surroundings? Are there sounds? Sensations? Are there scents in the air?

If this is a moment of shared kindness with others, do we recall facial expressions or body language, or do we hear a comforting tone of voice?

Let's continue immersing ourselves in this nourishing moment for a minute or so.

Having connected with this nurturing resource, let's now bring attention to our body in the present moment, noticing sensations and feelings. Has anything shifted? If we find pleasant or neutral sensations, such as a warmth in the chest, relaxation of the shoulders, a smile on the face, we may rest with those. If instead we notice areas of discomfort, we may take a few breaths to settle the body and mind, or direct our attention back to the nurturing resource for a few moments, or shift our attention to a different part of the body that feels better.

Finally, let's reflect: How important are such moments of comfort and safety for our well-being?

And how important are acts of kindness and compassion to create a safe and secure world where our fellow human beings can thrive?

Seeing the value of kindness and compassion, how might that shift our perspective on our own life and our relationships with others?

Let's dedicate our practice today to those we know to be in need of health and well-being and, as we are able, expand this dedication to include a widening circle of beings on this earth.

And let's conclude by setting an intention to extend the skills and insights from this practice into everyday life.

Melancholy, Medicine, and the Transition

It's often hard to know if what you're experiencing requires an antidepressant, HT, a thyroid supplement, or vitamin and mineral supplements. Intractable sadness, irritability, sleeplessness, and more can be signs of any of these things. If you've had depression before you can be more vulnerable now. In a moment when you won't feel ready, you'll have to take charge of getting the right tests and tracking symptoms when you take anything new. You'll need to be proactive about working with your doctor to make adjustments to doses of antidepressants and hormones. During the Transition and in the Upgrade, ask for these tests:

- Thyroid: TSH, free-T4-to-T3 conversion
- Vitamin and mineral levels: vitamin B_{12}, vitamin D
- Post-Transition: free estrogen, free testosterone, and DHEA-S

Keep a log of how you feel when you start taking something new. Often something that is supposed to help can make you feel worse.

If you do start an antidepressant or HT, ask your doctor for forms that can allow you to track your dose to find your own sweet spot.

Remember that the simplest way to know if you've hit the Transition is by seeing that your cycle shortens by one or more days two or more times in a year.

Tracking Your Moods: How to Make a Log

Make a few columns for time of day, ideally morning, afternoon, and evening, to track mood on a 1–10 scale: Am I feeling happy (10) or sad (1)? Optimistic (10) or pessimistic (1)? Also three times a day, note energy or a feeling of zest for life on a scale of 1 to 10, 10 being totally engaged and energetic. Track mental clarity an hour before and two hours after taking any progestin or SSRI, 10 being super clear, 1 a total fog. Also track libido daily (raring to go being 10; "Are you kidding?" being 1), note how frequently you feel hot or sweaty, and in the morning, write about your quality of sleep the night before. How many times did you wake? How long did it take to go back to sleep? How many times were you hot or sweaty? Note the time and dose of all medications and supplements so you can see if they are interacting or if any of them might be at the root of some overwhelming good or bad feelings. Having your journal as hard evidence of your mood prior to taking hormones or medication can be a lifesaver.

After the first few visits, I tracked with my patients the top three issues for them weekly, noting how they characterized them. For example, brain fog, lack of joy, irritability, anxiety, insomnia, tearfulness, anger, depression, and so forth. Because I was able to see what they kept track of it was much easier for me to adjust medication each time in a way that was more targeted to their actual individual symptoms. Remember: NSAIDs can block SSRIs's effectiveness. When you've charted these things for six to eight weeks, you can figure out what is going on and have data to help you adjust the dosage accordingly. With most of my patients, we'd find their new sweet spot after about three to six months. With this kind of information in hand, you have a better chance of making it happen sooner.

The Tricky World of Supplements

Check manufacturers of supplements for independent testing. Supplements are not regulated, and they don't always contain what's advertised. And beware the hype, since no FDA approval is required to make sure they do what they claim to do.

Vitamins and supplements can interact with one another, with your prescription drugs, and with your OTC drugs. And you may have sensitivities that are unexpected. Many women tell me they take a quarter of what's recommended and that suits them just fine. You'll need help from a qualified professional to figure out what works and what doesn't. This area is still new and under-researched, so be ready to sort through conflicting advice.

As with all medicines, keep a log of symptoms for everything new that you take. Some things that are meant to make you feel better can make you feel worse. For example, some probiotics can cause brain fog. Don't be quick to blame symptoms on stress or on the way the stars are aligned. It might be that new substance causing the problem.

My approach in general is that less is more, so I stay away from taking too many things preventively. *Harvard Women's Health Watch* warns for example that calcium supplements may make some women as much as seven times more likely to develop dementia, and we are already at higher risk in later years. If it ain't broke, don't fix it. Keep the pill popping to a minimum. (With all the hype I know that's hard.)

Taking Charge of Your Prescriptions: Checking the Beers Criteria Anticholinergic Scale

It happens like this: You visit a doctor to resolve reflux and are given medication for it. Then you hurt your arm and start taking an NSAID. Your stomach gets upset and you get medicine for that as well. Side effects pile up and symptom whack-a-mole snowballs with more medication. You get foggy and disoriented, and another doctor decides it's dementia because in tests your cognitive levels have clearly declined. This problem, polypharmacy, has to stop. And it may rest on your shoulders to stop it.

Every visit to the doctor has to include a review of all medication and supplements. Take a complete list of all your pills, patches, creams, and supplements. You can start your own review by researching a few scales, including the Anticholinergic Cognitive Burden, the Drug Burden Index–sedative component, and the Drug Burden Index–anticholinergic component, as well as the Beers criteria for inappropriate medications.

Remember, choline is needed for healthy brain function. Many drugs are anticholinergic, including those given for incontinence. Incontinence in many cases can be resolved through physical activity and physical therapy. See "The Vagina Gym" below.

When Common Conditions Are Mistaken for Dementia

If you or a loved one seems to be sliding quickly into strong cognitive decline, check these common conditions before jumping to conclusions about dementia. These are conditions in which disorientation and memory loss can be corrected.

- Urinary tract infections: As we age, we don't feel the symptoms as strongly, the burning and discomfort from peeing. The infection doesn't get caught as quickly, and in the body's effort to fight it, there will be inflammation throughout the body and brain that can cause cognitive issues. An antibiotic can clear this up within days.

- Urinary retention: If you just started a new medication and you can't pee or you find it a struggle, this could be an anticholinergic effect, and cognitive impact may be a simultaneous symptom. This can even be caused by taking high doses of Tylenol recommended by a doctor for pain after a procedure or surgery.

- Depression: Symptoms of disorientation may seem like dementia, but they may instead be signs of early clinical depression. An SSRI or SNRI may clear the confusion caused by depression.

- Drug or alcohol side effects, particularly the anticholinergic side effects of many drugs discussed above.

- Subdural hematoma: Did you hit your head and now find yourself losing your balance easily or sitting a bit lopsided? It could be a brain bruise, which is easier to develop as we age. Get to the doctor and have it checked. This is nothing to mess around with. It can be reversed if caught soon enough.

- Normal pressure hydrocephalus (NPH): This happens when extra spinal fluid seeps into the crevices of the brain but doesn't raise intracranial pressure. The excess fluid can interrupt brain function. It can be treated by placing a simple shunt to drain the excess fluid.

Eat Your Way to an Upgrade

There are a lot of crazy, extreme diets out there, but over time, two principles for optimal nutrition have held true: the Mediterranean diet and meal timing.

Intermittent Fasting: It's All in the Timing

Cleo, fifty-one, had been running for years. She ran ten miles daily—if she couldn't schedule a single long run, she ran to and from work, five miles each way. She was always a healthy eater, but somehow she kept gaining weight, and the mental fog just wouldn't lift. She'd been thin all her life and she was now thirty-five pounds overweight. She was getting sadder by the minute. She didn't know if it was body image or something else that was making her feel so down.

Humans did not evolve eating three big meals and two snacks a day around a fire. They were kinetic, always on the move, they were grazers, and they probably weren't overweight. Emerging evidence shows that eating all your daily calories within an eight-hour window, making sure there are at least twelve to sixteen hours between dinner and breakfast, is great for metabolism and in promoting brain health. The reason for extending daily fasting is to mobilize your body fat to be metabolized. When you don't eat, your insulin goes down. The liver's glycogen reserves are available as fuel for the brain for only twelve hours after your last meal. When that runs out, the brain turns to using stored fat in other parts of the body for fuel. The brain doesn't have its own fat, so it prompts the body to break down fat and transport it through the blood supply.

On the advice of a nutritionist, Cleo began intermittent fasting (IF) combined with a Mediterranean diet. She started eating two big meals a day—and one snack: waiting until noon for her first and finishing dinner by 7:30 P.M.—and if she was headed out for an extra-long morning run, she would have a spoonful of nut butter and a small cappuccino beforehand. Not only did she lose the thirty-five pounds, but her brain fog lifted. "The weight melted off," she said, "and I feel sharp and alert again. Like my old self." Researchers at MIT found that this approach stimulates neural stem cells, which are key for replacing old, worn-out cells—keeping your brain resilient and flexible. And it has been shown to help you lose more fat and retain the muscle that triggers the brain to keep cognition, emotion, and judgment at peak levels.

Leaving twelve to sixteen hours between dinner and breakfast stresses the metabolism in the way that weights and exercise stress your heart and muscles in order to strengthen them. A little bit of metabolic stress from fasting can end up making your cells and tissues stronger and more resistant to disease. And anything that reduces chronic inflammation makes the gut-brain team function at its best. That in turn improves a range of health issues from arthritic pain to asthma, while lowering the risk for cancers by clearing toxins and damaged cells

Pack On the Protein

One last piece of the puzzle is protein. You know by now that movement and cognition are linked, and muscle strength is key to remaining active. Protein is the nutritional key to maintaining muscle, which in turn helps us keep our clarity and memory and lifts our mood.

As we age, we lose muscle strength faster, so you actually need to eat *more* protein than when you were younger. It is estimated that 41 percent of adult women have dietary protein intakes below the recommended daily allowance (RDA). In a 2018 study that followed more than 2,900 people over sixty-five for more than twenty-three years, researchers found that those who ate the most protein were 30 percent less likely to become functionally impaired than those who ate the lowest amount. Even if you have to drink it, get your protein intake up to between 60 and 90 grams per day, depending on your size. It will take planning to get that much into your diet. You'll need to save room and calories for that second piece of fish at lunch or dinner.

Healthy Microbiome: Honoring the Gut Brain

Keeping inflammation in check means a healthier microbiome. Too much sugar/carbs causes inflammation, and researchers around the world are learning that artificial sweeteners might be even worse. Most of the sweeteners—including natural forms like stevia and birch xylitol—cause alterations in the microbiome, creating an environment for the growth of unhealthy bacteria that can invade the bloodstream. Sugar substitutes can also send signals to activate the brain's dopamine circuits. This is the intense pleasure/reward system; overstimulation is the mechanism at the heart of addiction. Satisfying the cravings in turn can trigger glucose intolerance, making us crave more sugar, setting up the condition that leads to diabetes. Diabetes, or prediabetes, equals chronic inflammation. Chronic inflammation equals brain shrinkage. Brain shrinkage equals cognitive decline: a downgrade, not an Upgrade.

Eating too much; eating high-salt fast foods, low-fiber foods, fried foods, trans fats, sugars, or chemical additives in processed foods; nicotine; drinking alcohol; poor sleep quality; and being sedentary can all destroy the healthy microbiome. If we are having carb cravings, it could mean we don't have friendly bacteria signaling contentment to the brain, and so the quickest way to remedy that is to goose the brain into boosting the feel-good chemicals, dopamine and serotonin, which are most easily triggered by sugars. The high doesn't last long, and pretty soon we are either exhausted on the couch or reaching for caffeine or another candy bar. It's a vicious cycle that disables the all-important gut brain.

Add to the list antibiotics and laxatives; even the chlorine and fluoride found in some tap water can be dangerous to the microbiome. Chlorine evaporates after a while at room temperature, but you can boil your water to remove it more quickly. Treasure your microbiome. Feed and cultivate it carefully. Work with your specialist to find the right fermented foods and/or probiotic for you if your microbiome needs repopulating.

Actionable Numbers on Inflammation

Your doctor can help you gather the information you need to understand how much work you might have to do to battle inflammation and preserve health and cognition. Here are some markers to track via blood work and genetic testing that can help you make good decisions on diet and supplements:

- Heart: A calcium scan can help you understand how much animal fat you can eat and if you need a statin.

- Brain: Check for the APOE4 gene variation to make an informed decision about HT. If you have even one mutation and have a family history of dementia, it might influence you to add estrogen during the Transition, since we know it can protect cognition.
- Hemoglobin A1C, C-reactive protein, triglycerides, LDL, VLDL (very low-density lipids): These tests can indicate diabetes, heart and vascular issues, and general "zombie-cell" inflammation. If any of these numbers is off, cut the sugars/carbs/unhealthy fats and emphasize lean protein and nonstarchy vegetables. Consider a statin if LDL is over 100.
- Hemoglobin, hematocrit, and red blood cell width: If you have heavy bleeding during the Transition, it's very likely you're anemic. Most doctors check hemoglobin and hematocrit levels to determine whether or not you need an iron supplement. But there is another test, red blood cell width, that indicates whether or not the bone marrow has caught up in red blood cell production. That measurement will tell you if your anemia is actually resolved.

Remember, the body's inflammation goes higher naturally with age, so it's more important than ever, if you want an Upgraded brain, to keep inflammation under control. The keys to doing this are:

- Getting enough sleep
- Exercising to exhilaration, not exhaustion
- Relying on nonstarchy vegetables and lean protein for most of your nutrition
- Avoiding alcohol, sugar, too much salt, fried foods, and overeating and overexercising

Be alert to new discoveries. They used to tell you not to eat eggs. Now eggs are considered a source of healthy omegas and their yolks a particularly good source of choline (great for the brain). That gets confusing. On Monday you hear A; on Friday you hear not A. Both could be true, because A will work for one woman while it will harm another. What has panned out over time is what I have emphasized here, though keep watching for new and helpful markers that are beginning to come into sight.

The Vagina Gym

In other news of adjustments down there during the Transition, if you've had babies and/or pelvic surgery, you're probably familiar with the panic that comes just before a cough or a sneeze, or the moment you have to run to catch a green light or a bus. *How much pee is going to come out? A little drop, or a noticeable squirt?* "I just can't bring myself to buy Depends or Poise pads," says Christina, sixty-five, who still runs to try to keep the post-Transition weight off. After three kids she is having trouble holding her pee. "It makes me feel too old to buy anything in the incontinence aisle, so I use maxi pads." Christina, however, is on her third round of antibiotics for a stubborn urinary tract infection. It's not a surprise. Pads for your period are designed to hold a lot less liquid. If you use menstrual pads, the urine will overwhelm the pad's capacity and the liquid will stay close to your skin. Can you say "middle-aged diaper rash"? Christina's recurring UTIs are most likely being made worse by not using the right equipment.

Christina doesn't want to change her habits, but targeted exercises like those in a barre class will help tone the pelvic floor and help her hold her pee. Pelvic floor physical therapy—and yes, sometimes it means they manipulate muscles from inside the vagina—can cure the problem for some women. When I broach the subject with her, she wants neither. "I hate barre classes. Running keeps me thinner. And I'm not letting anyone poke around down there unless I have to let them."

Insistence on running while not addressing pelvic floor issues or not remaining sexually active also can be a recipe for prolapse of the vagina, the rectum, the bladder, the uterus. This happens more often than you think, and women sometimes wait years before telling their doctor they are having a problem. Meanwhile, these issues can destroy a woman's confidence and intimate life, putting her at risk of depression. She doesn't want surgery, which entails pinning organs back into place, even though the results—putting you back into social settings you've been afraid to enter—are life-changing. So get it fixed if other things haven't worked!

You have choices in how you meet changes like this. You can fight them, resist them, deny what's happening, hide them from everyone, and take the well-trodden path to a downgrade. Or you can turn to face the road less traveled, work with what you have, and create the conditions for making this time of your life an Upgrade. We have agency. Peeing when you sneeze is not inevitable. How our destiny unfolds is up to us.

Estrogen builds thickness and lubrication in mucous membranes, so as estrogen declines, so will vaginal lubrication. Even with HT it might be time to break out the lube, like Slippery Stuff, and you may need vaginal estrogen cream. And wash the minute you are done. The skin is more sensitive to small tears, and as men age and their semen becomes more acidic, your body will like it less. You'll be much more prone to UTIs. Yes, this will all take away some spontaneity, but it's better than nothing. Find a way to make a game of it.

If you're having trouble with vaginal dryness or painful intercourse, estrogen inserted up to twice weekly can be super helpful. You'll find it in the form of a cream like Estrace, Estring, Vagifem, and others, or in vaginal suppositories or rings. Ask your primary doctor or ob-gyn for a prescription. The upside of vaginal insertion is that these forms of HT have been shown to be safe even for women with a breast cancer risk.

Supportive Modalities for the Upgrade

We know you'll find your own way to support movement, nutrition, and nervous-system maintenance for the Upgrade, but people I trust have found a few things that have been helpful. I can't guarantee results, and you'll have to monitor your own risks, but maybe here's a start:

- **Nutrition and cognitive change:** Noom, a weight-loss app, has been helpful in shifting attitudes toward food and health and sustaining healthy diet, exercise, and emotional habits.

  If you just want a weight, nutrition, and calorie counter, Lose It! is a great app for that.

- **Exercise for pelvic floor strength, joint lubrication, and core strength:** Xtend Barre classes on the Openfit app. Many of the other programs on Openfit may be a bit too intense, but Xtend Barre, XB Pilates, and XB Stretch have great basics for fitness and for strengthening our weakest parts.

  Since many of us are more sedentary than we think, getting a Fitbit or an Apple Watch and using the activity app will give great feedback on how much you're moving and how many calories you're actually burning through exercise, as opposed to what you think you're burning. Yes, most of us overestimate, eat more than we burn, and then decide that exercise doesn't help us lose weight.

- **Nervous-system maintenance and conscious Upgrading:**
  Body scans: These relaxation techniques are great for destressing, resetting, and sleeping. There are many to be found on YouTube, Netflix, Spotify, and Apple Podcasts. Headspace or Calm is a good place to begin if you've never done anything like this before.

  Learning to focus: Concentration meditation is different from relaxation. We're not looking to just calm; we are also looking to sharpen, train, and steady the mind. Once we accomplish that, we can start to focus on change and developing the qualities we've always wanted to have as the woman we've always wanted to be. The compassion protocol in the next paragraph also has great training for steadying the mind.

  Cultivating compassion: Emory University has developed a protocol that does it all: calms the nervous system, steadies the mind, helps you find compassion for yourself, and teaches you to develop compassion that energizes, keeping you from burning out from the world's grief.

For help dealing with long-haul Covid brain fog issues: Visit https://www.verywellhealth.com/dealing-with-covid-brain-fog-5209460.

For help dealing with teen or adult children who struggle with addiction or mental health issues, Al-anon has an excellent twelve step program for parents: Visit www.al-anon.org and search for "parents programs".

Acknowledgments

This book had its beginnings when several fans of *The Female Brain* reached out to me and wondered if I would please do a book on the next phase of a woman's life, after fertility and into the years of empowerment and wisdom. At first I was skeptical, since all the medical science focused only on what goes wrong in the second half, but I realized that no one had yet mapped out these stages of development for women. So here it is, *The Upgrade,* and I have so many to thank for what I have learned, what I am becoming every day. To anyone I missed, you know who you are: thank you.

I want to thank my UCSF colleagues, supporters, and mentors: Cori Bargmann, Lynne Krillich Benioff, Marc Benioff, Liz Blackburn, Jennifer Cummings, Mary Dallman, Alison Doupe, Dena Dubal, Elissa Epel, Laura Esserman, Adam Gazzaley, Anna Glezer, Mindy Goldman, Lyn Gracie, Mel Grumbach, Steve Hauser, Dixie Honig, Holly Ingraham, Cynthia Kenyon, Joel Kramer, Rob Malenka, Sindy Mellon, Michael Merzenich, Bruce Miller, Nancy Milliken, Tammy Neuhouse, Thomas C. Neylan, Kim Norman, Faina Novosolov, Aoife O'Donovan, Christina Pham, Ricki Pollycove, Sandy Robertson, John Rubenstein, Alla Spivak, Brandon Staglin, Garen Staglin, Shari Staglin, Matt State, Marc Tessier-Lavigne, Owen Wolkowitz, and Kristine Yaffe.

I want to thank my UC Berkeley teachers, mentors, and colleagues, especially Frank Beach, Marian Diamond, Peter Hornick, Daniel Mazia, Clyde Willson, and Fred Wilt.

I want to thank my Yale teachers, mentors, and colleagues, especially Marilyn Farquar, Florence Hazeltine, Stanley Jackson, Eric Nestler, Sherwin Nuland and Philip Sarrel.

I want to thank my UC London and Wellcome Institute teachers, mentors, and colleagues, especially Bill Bynum, Charlotte MacKenzie, Roy Porter, Janet Thompson, and Richard Wollheim.

I want to thank my Harvard teachers, mentors, and colleagues, especially Mary Anne Badaraco, Myron Belfer, Beth Blessing, Herb Goldings, Kathy Kelly, William Meissner, George Valliant, Bessel van der Kolk, and Peggy Wingard.

I want to thank my other colleagues in the women's neuroscience field, especially Roberta Brinton, John Cacioppo, Larry Cahill, Lee Cohen, Neill Epperson, Stephani Faubion, Jill Goldstein, Jennifer Gordon, Victor Henderson, Melissa Hines, Sarah Hrdy, Hadine Joffe, Claudia Kawas, Eleanor Maccoby, Martha McClintock, Bruce McEwen, Pauline Maki, Lisa Mosconi, Barbara Parry, Jennifer Payne, Natalie Rasgon, David Rubinow, Peter Schmidt, Barbara Sherwin, and Deborah Tannen and Myrna Weissman.

I want to thank my friends who keep me going in my own Upgrade: my Saturday girlfriend lunch gang: Jennifer Curley, Mickey Berg Kordelos, Lin Repola, Glenda Seidel, Maria Carini Sneed, and Marty Wolf; my women's dinner group gang: Kimberely Cameron Brody, Maggie Cox, Juannie Eng, Katherine Honig, Kerry King, Sandy Kleiman, Susan Lopes, Kary Schulman, and Brenda Way; my Mill Valley photography group; my go-to writers: Julie Margaret Hogben, Jena Pincot, and Michelle Stacey; my Mill Valley meditation group; my Jewel Heart meditation teachers and group; my aquatics class teachers and teammates, Patricia Chytrowski, Peggy Conrad, Kathy King, Suzanne Paynovich, and Marianne Wilman; my girlfriends who always pick up the phone when I call: Diane Cirrincione, Alice Corning, Jean Hietpas, Lisa Klairmont, Adrienne Larkin, Sharon Agopian Melodia, Sue Rosen, Wendy Shearn, Mary Sherman,

Nancy Todes-Taylor, and Jody Yeary; my mother's dearest girlfriend from childhood, Caroline "Maury" Knight, who has shared some juicy stories; and my dear friend the late Janet Durant.

I want to thank my literary team at Harmony; my wonderful editor Donna Loffredo, whose skills have made this book what it is; my agent, Elizabeth Kaplan, whose dedication, availability, and advice have been everything I could hope for and more.

And a big shout-out and thank-you to all the fans of *The Female Brain* for your support, letters, and questions over the years. With every letter and question you have challenged me to hear different voices, to learn more so I can become more helpful along our Upgrading path.

I would like to thank my family, especially my sister Diana Brizendine, who supports me every day with her love and prayers, my loving son John Whitney Brizendine, whose support and lightning-fast computer skills helped me finish this book. And to my brother Buzz Brizendine, in memory of my sister Paula Brizendine Kuntz, my stepdaughters Jessica and Elizabeth Barondes, uncles Tom and John Brizendine and aunts Kath and Shirl Brizendine, and nieces Jessica Johns, Morgan Brizendine, Rachel Llanes, Nicole Kuntz, and Louisa Llanes, and nephews Ryan Brizendine and Derek Kuntz who cheered me on. The memory of my mother, Louise Ann Brizendine, who is with me every day and knew what was important in life.

I would like to thank my husband, Samuel Barondes, whose love, wisdom, and support keep me going. He is my gem.

It's hard to put into words my appreciation and gratitude to my writing partner, editor, and friend Amy Hertz, whose professional skills, talent, and breadth as a person have challenged and guided me through the process of writing not only *The Upgrade* but also *The Female Brain*. Without her neither of these books would have come to fruition.

I especially want to thank all those patients whose stories I told but who, for confidentiality reasons, must remain anonymous. Their struggles and joys in Upgrading are gifted to you to help guide you in your own Upgrade.

Selected References

Author's Note

Davis, Emily J., Iryna Lobach, and Dena B. Dubal. 2018. "Female XX sex chromosomes increase survival and extend lifespan in aging mice." *Aging Cell* 18 (1). doi: 10.1111/acel.12871.

Santoro, Nanette, and John F. Randolph. 2011. "Reproductive hormones and the menopause transition." *Obstetrics and Gynecology Clinics of North America* 38 (3):455–66. doi: 10.1016/j.ogc.2011.05.004.

Sripada, Rebecca K., Christine E. Marx, Anthony P. King, Nirmala Rajaram, Sarah N. Garfinkel, James L. Abelson, and Israel Liberzon. 2013. "DHEA enhances emotion regulation neurocircuits and modulates memory for emotional stimuli." *Neuropsychopharmacology* 38 (9):1798–1807. doi: 10.1038/npp.2013.79.

Taylor, Caitlin M., Laura Pritschet, and Emily G. Jacobs. 2021. "The scientific body of knowledge—whose body does it serve? A spotlight on oral contraceptives and women's health factors in neuroimaging." *Frontiers in Neuroendocrinology* 60 (6). doi: 10.1016/j.yfrne.2020.100874.

Chapter 1: Changing the Conversation

Archer, John. 2019. "The reality and evolutionary significance of human psychological sex differences." *Biological Reviews* 94 (4):1381–415. doi: 10.1111/brv.12507.

Luine, Victoria, and Maya Frankfurt. 2020. "Estrogenic regulation of memory: The first 50 years." *Hormones and Behavior* 121. doi: 10.1016/j.yhbeh.2020.104711.

Monteleone, Patrizia, Giulia Mascagni, Andrea Giannini, Andrea R. Genazzani, and Tommaso Simoncini. 2018. "Symptoms of menopause—global prevalence, physiology and implications." *Nature Reviews Endocrinology* 14 (4):199–215. doi: 10.1038/nrendo.2017.180.

Protsenko, Ekaterina, Ruoting Yang, Brent Nier, Victor Reus, Rasha Hammamieh, Ryan Rampersaud, et al. 2021. "'GrimAge,' an epigenetic predictor of mortality, is accelerated in major depressive disorder." *Translational Psychiatry* 11 (1). doi: 10.1038/s41398-021-01302-0.

Sartori, Andrea C., David E. Vance, Larry Z. Slater, and Michael Crowe. 2012. "The impact of inflammation on cognitive function in older adults." *Journal of Neuroscience Nursing* 44 (4):206–17. doi: 10.1097/JNN.0b013e3182527690.

Torréns, Javier I., Kim Sutton-Tyrrell, Xinhua Zhao, Karen Matthews, Sarah Brockwell, MaryFran Sowers, and Nanette Santoro. 2009. "Relative androgen excess during the menopausal transition predicts incident metabolic syndrome in midlife women." *Menopause* 16 (2):257–64. doi: 10.1097/gme.0b013e318185e249.

Wang, Yiwei, Aarti Mishra, and Roberta Diaz Brinton. 2020. "Transitions in metabolic and immune systems from pre-menopause to post-menopause: Implications for age-associated neurodegenerative diseases." *F1000Research* 9. doi: 10.12688/f1000research.21599.1.

Xin, Jiang, Yaoxue Zhang, Yan Tang, and Yuan Yang. 2019. "Brain differences between men and women: Evidence from deep learning." *Frontiers in Neuroscience* 13. doi: 10.3389/fnins.2019.00185.

Chapter 2: The Crux of Being Female

Hill, Sarah. *This Is Your Brain on Birth Control: The Surprising Science of Sex, Women, Hormones, and the Law of Unintended Consequences*. New York: Penguin, 2019.

Mueller, Joshua M., Laura Pritschet, Tyler Santander, Caitlin M. Taylor, Scott T. Grafton, Emily Goard Jacobs, and Jean M. Carlson. 2021. "Dynamic community detection reveals transient reorganization of functional brain networks across a female menstrual cycle." *Network Neuroscience* 5 (1):125–44. doi: 10.1162/netn_a_00169.

Paul, Steven M., Graziano Pinna, and Alessandro Guidotti. 2020. "Allopregnanolone: From molecular pathophysiology to therapeutics. A historical perspective." *Neurobiology of Stress* 12. doi: 10.1016/j.ynstr.2020.100215.

Pritschet, Laura, Tyler Santander, Caitlin M. Taylor, Evan Layher, Shuying Yu, Michael B. Miller, et al. 2020. "Functional reorganization of brain networks across the human menstrual cycle." *NeuroImage* 220 (4). doi: 10.1016/j. neuroimage.2020.117091.

Syan, Sabrina K., Luciano Minuzzi, Dustin Costescu, Mara Smith, Olivia R. Allega, Marg Coote, et al. 2017. "Influence of endogenous estradiol, progesterone, allopregnanolone, and dehydroepiandrosterone sulfate on brain resting state functional connectivity across the menstrual cycle." *Fertility and Sterility* 107 (5):1246–55.e4. doi: 10.1016/j.fertnstert.2017.03.021.

Weber, Miriam T., Mark Mapstone, Jennifer Staskiewicz, and Pauline M. Maki. 2012. "Reconciling subjective memory complaints with objective memory performance in the menopausal transition." *Menopause* 19 (7):735–41. doi: 10.1097/gme.0b013e318241fd22.

Witchel, Selma Feldman, Bianca Pinto, Anne Claire Burghard, and Sharon E. Oberfield. 2020. "Update on adrenarche." *Current Opinion in Pediatrics* 32 (4):574–81. doi: 10.1097/mop.0000000000000928.

Chapter 3: Transitioning into the Upgrade

Bluming, Avrum Z. 2021. "Progesterone and breast cancer pathogenesis." *Journal of Molecular Endocrinology* 66 (1):C1–C2. doi: 10.1530/jme-20-0262.

Boyle, Christina P., Cyrus A. Raji, Kirk I. Erickson, Oscar L. Lopez, James T. Becker, H. Michael Gach, et al. 2020. "Estrogen, brain structure, and cognition in postmenopausal women." *Human Brain Mapping* 42 (1):24–35. doi: 10.1002/hbm.25200.

Craig, A. D., K. Chen, D. Bandy, and E. M. Reiman. 2000. "Thermosensory activation of insular cortex." *Nature Neuroscience* 3 (2):184–90. doi: 10.1038/72131.

El Khoudary, Samar R., Gail Greendale, Sybil L. Crawford, Nancy E. Avis, Maria M. Brooks, Rebecca C. Thurston, et al. 2019. "The menopause transition and women's health at midlife." *Menopause* 26 (10):1213–27. doi: 10.1097/gme.0000000000001424.

Engel, Sinha, Hannah Klusmann, Beate Ditzen, Christine Knaevelsrud, and Sarah Schumacher. 2019. "Menstrual cycle-related fluctuations in oxytocin concentrations: A systematic review and meta-analysis." *Frontiers in Neuroendocrinology* 52 (6):144–55. doi: 10.1016/j.yfrne.2018.11.002.

Fan, Yubo, Ruiyi Tang, Jerilynn C. Prior, and Rong Chen. 2020. "Paradigm shift in pathophysiology of vasomotor symptoms: Effects of estradiol withdrawal and progesterone therapy." *Drug Discovery Today: Disease Models* 32 (1):59–69. doi: 10.1016/j.ddmod.2020.11.004.

Freedman, Robert R. 2014. "Menopausal hot flashes: Mechanisms, endocrinology, treatment." *Journal of Steroid Biochemistry and Molecular Biology* 142:115–20. doi: 10.1016/j.jsbmb.2013.08.010.

Goldstein, S. R., and M. A. Lumsden. 2017. "Abnormal uterine bleeding in perimenopause." *Climacteric* 20 (5):414–20. doi: 10.1080/13697137.2017.1358921.

Hanstede, Miriam M. F., Martijn J. Burger, Anne Timmermans, and Matthé P. M Burger. 2012. "Regional and temporal variation in hysterectomy rates and surgical routes for benign diseases in the Netherlands." *Acta Obstetricia et Gynecologica Scandinavica* 91 (2):220–25. doi: 10.1111/j.1600-0412.2011.01309.x.

Henderson, V. W., J. R. Guthrie, E. C. Dudley, H. G. Burger, and L. Dennerstein. 2003. "Estrogen exposures and memory at midlife: A population-based study of women." *Neurology* 60 (8):1369–71. doi: 10.1212/01.Wnl.0000059413.75888.Be.

Hodis, H. N., and P. M. Sarrel. 2018. "Menopausal hormone therapy and breast cancer: what is the evidence from randomized trials?" *Climacteric* 21 (6):521–28. doi: 10.1080/13697137.2018.1514008.

Nanba, Aya T., Juilee Rege, Jianwei Ren, Richard J. Auchus, William E. Rainey, and Adina F. Turcu. 2019. "11-Oxygenated C19 steroids do not decline with age in women." *Journal of Clinical Endocrinology & Metabolism* 104 (7):2615–22. doi: 10.1210/jc.2018-02527.

Pletzer, Belinda, Ti-Anni Harris, Andrea Scheuringer, and Esmeralda Hidalgo-Lopez. 2019. "The cycling brain: Menstrual cycle related fluctuations in hippocampal and fronto-striatal activation and connectivity during cognitive tasks." *Neuropsychopharmacology* 44 (11):1867–75. doi: 10.1038/s41386-019-0435-3.

Pouba, Katherine, and Ashley Tianen. 2006. "Lunacy in the 19th Century: Women's Admission to Asylums in the United States of America." *Oshkosh Scholar* 1:95–103.

Santoro, Nanette, and John F. Randolph. 2011. "Reproductive hormones and the menopause transition." *Obstetrics and Gynecology Clinics of North America* 38 (3):455–66. doi: 10.1016/j.ogc.2011.05.004.

Süss, Hannah, Jasmine Willi, Jessica Grub, and Ulrike Ehlert. 2021. "Estradiol and progesterone as resilience markers?—Findings from the Swiss Perimenopause Study." *Psychoneuroendocrinology* 127. doi: 10.1016/j.psyneuen.2021.105177.

Taylor, Caitlin M., Laura Pritschet, and Emily G. Jacobs. 2021. "The scientific body of knowledge—whose body does it serve? A spotlight on oral contraceptives and women's health factors in neuroimaging." *Frontiers in Neuroendocrinology* 60. doi: 10.1016/j.yfrne.2020.100874.

Weber, M. T., L. H. Rubin, R. Schroeder, T. Steffenella, and P. M. Maki. 2021. "Cognitive profiles in perimenopause: Hormonal and menopausal symptom correlates." *Climacteric* 24 (4):1–7. doi: 10.1080/13697137.2021.1892626.

Zorumski, Charles F., Steven M. Paul, Douglas F. Covey, and Steven Mennerick. 2019. "Neurosteroids as novel antidepressants and anxiolytics: GABA-A receptors and beyond." *Neurobiology of Stress* 11. doi: 10.1016/j.ynstr.2019.100196.

Chapter 4: Navigating the Wilderness

Allais, Gianni, Giulia Chiarle, Silvia Sinigaglia, Gisella Airola, Paola Schiapparelli, and Chiara Benedetto. 2018. "Estrogen, migraine, and vascular risk." *Neurological Sciences* 39 (S1):11–20. doi: 10.1007/s10072-018-3333-2.

Beral, Valerie, Richard Peto, Kirstin Pirie, and Gillian Reeves. 2019. "Type and timing of menopausal hormone therapy and breast cancer risk: individual participant meta-analysis of the worldwide epidemiological evidence." *The Lancet* 394 (10204):1159–68. doi: 10.1016/s0140-6736(19)31709-x.

Brinton, Roberta Diaz, Richard F. Thompson, Michael R. Foy, Michel Baudry, JunMing Wang, Caleb E. Finch, et al. 2008. "Progesterone receptors: Form and function in brain." *Frontiers in Neuroendocrinology* 29 (2):313–39. doi: 10.1016/j.yfrne.2008.02.001.

Bromberger, Joyce T., and Cynthia Neill Epperson. 2018. "Depression during and after the perimenopause." *Obstetrics and Gynecology Clinics of North America* 45 (4):663–78. doi: 10.1016/j.ogc.2018.07.007.

Cagnacci, Angelo, and Martina Venier. 2019. "The controversial history of hormone replacement therapy." *Medicina* 55 (9). doi: 10.3390/medicina55090602.

Cummings, Jennifer A., and Louann Brizendine. 2002. "Comparison of physical and emotional side effects of progesterone or medroxyprogesterone in early postmenopausal women." *Menopause* 9 (4):253–63. doi: 10.1097/00042192-200207000-00006.

"Dietary Supplements: What You Need to Know." National Institutes of Health Office of Dietary Supplements, September 3, 2020.

Edwards, Alexis C., Sara Larsson Lönn, Casey Crump, Eve K. Mościcki, Jan Sundquist, Kenneth S. Kendler, and Kristina Sundquist. 2020. "Oral contraceptive use and risk of suicidal behavior among young women." *Psychological Medicine*:1–8. doi: 10.1017/s0033291720003475.

Genazzani, Andrea R., Patrizia Monteleone, Andrea Giannini, and Tommaso Simoncini. 2021. "Hormone therapy in the postmenopausal years: considering benefits and risks in clinical practice." *Human Reproduction Update* doi: 10.1093/humupd/dmab026.

Gibson, Carolyn J., Yixia Li, Guneet K. Jasuja, Kyle J. Self, Karen H. Seal, and Amy L. Byers. 2021. "Menopausal hormone therapy and suicide in a national sample of midlife and older women veterans." *Medical Care* 59:S70–S76. doi: 10.1097/mlr.0000000000001433.

Gordon, Jennifer L., Tory A. Eisenlohr-Moul, David R. Rubinow, Leah Schrubbe, and Susan S. Girdler. 2016. "Naturally occurring changes in estradiol concentrations in the menopause transition predict morning cortisol and negative mood in perimenopausal depression." *Clinical Psychological Science* 4 (5):919–35. doi: 10.1177/2167702616647924.

Heath, Laura, Shelly L. Gray, Denise M. Boudreau, Ken Thummel, Karen L. Edwards, Stephanie M. Fullerton, et al. 2018. "Cumulative antidepressant use and risk of dementia in a prospective cohort study." *Journal of the American Geriatrics Society* 66 (10):1948–55. doi: 10.1111/jgs.15508.

Hill, Sarah. *This is Your Brain on Birth Control: The Surprising Science of Sex, Women, Hormones, and the law of Unintended Consequences.* New York: Penguin, 2019.

Kolata, Gina. "Rate of hysterectomies puzzles experts." *New York Times,* September 20, 1988.

Lobo, Roger A. 2016. "Hormone-replacement therapy: Current thinking." *Nature Reviews Endocrinology* 13 (4):220–31. doi: 10.1038/nrendo.2016.164.

Loprinzi, Charles L., Debra L. Barton, Lisa A. Carpenter, Jeff A. Sloan, Paul J. Novotny, Matthew T. Gettman, and Bradley J. Cristensen. 2004. "Pilot evaluation of paroxetine for treating hot flashes in men." *Mayo Clinic Proceedings* 79 (10):1247–51. doi: 10.4065/79.10.1247.

Maki, Pauline M., Susan G. Kornstein, Hadine Joffe, Joyce T. Bromberger, Ellen W. Freeman, Geena Athappilly, et al. 2019. "Guidelines for the evaluation and treatment of perimenopausal depression: Summary and recommendations." *Journal of Women's Health* 28 (2):117–34. doi: 10.1089/jwh.2018.27099.mensocrec.

Mazer, Norman A. 2004. "Interaction of estrogen therapy and thyroid hormone replacement in postmenopausal women." *Thyroid* 14 (S1):27–34. doi: 10.1089/105072504323024561.

Pokras, R., and V. G. Hufnagel. 1988. "Hysterectomy in the United States, 1965–84." *American Journal of Public Health* 78 (7):852–53. doi: 10.2105/ajph.78.7.852.

Rasgon, Natalie L., Jennifer Dunkin, Lynn Fairbanks, Lori L. Altshuler, Co Troung, Shana Elman, et al. 2007. "Estrogen and response to sertraline in postmenopausal women with major depressive disorder: A pilot study." *Journal of Psychiatric Research* 41 (3–4):338–43. doi: 10.1016/j.jpsychires.2006.03.009.

Russell, Jason K., Carrie K. Jones, and Paul A. Newhouse. 2019. "The role of estrogen in brain and cognitive aging." *Neurotherapeutics* 16 (3):649–65. doi: 10.1007/s13311-019-00766-9.

Singh, Meharvan, Chang Su, and Selena Ng. 2013. "Non-genomic mechanisms of progesterone action in the brain." *Frontiers in Neuroscience* 7. doi: 10.3389/fnins.2013.00159.

Skovlund, Charlotte Wessel, Lina Steinrud Mørch, Lars Vedel Kessing, Theis Lange, and Øjvind Lidegaard. 2018. "Association of hormonal contraception with suicide attempts and suicides." *American Journal of Psychiatry* 175 (4):336–42. doi: 10.1176/appi.ajp.2017.17060616.

Willi, Jasmine, Hannah Süss, Jessica Grub, and Ulrike Ehlert. 2020. "Prior depression affects the experience of the perimenopause—findings from the Swiss Perimenopause Study." *Journal of Affective Disorders* 277:603–11. doi: 10.1016/j.jad.2020.08.062.

Writing Group for the Women's Health Initiative, Investigators. 2002. "Risks and benefits of estrogen plus progestin in healthy postmenopausal women: principal results from the women's health initiative randomized controlled trial." *JAMA: The Journal of the American Medical Association* 288 (3):321–33. doi: 10.1001/jama.288.3.321.

Chapter 5: Renewal: Your Brain in Search of a New Reality

Freeman, Ellen W., Mary D. Sammel, David W. Boorman, and Rongmei Zhang. 2014. "Longitudinal pattern of depressive symptoms around natural menopause." *JAMA Psychiatry* 71 (1). doi: 10.1001/jamapsychiatry.2013.2819.

Gordon, Jennifer L., Alexis Peltier, Julia A. Grummisch, and Laurie Sykes Tottenham. 2019. "Estradiol fluctuation, sensitivity to stress, and depressive symptoms in the menopause transition: A pilot study." *Frontiers in Psychology* 10. doi: 10.3389/fpsyg.2019.01319.

Handa, Robert J., and Michael J. Weiser. 2014. "Gonadal steroid hormones and the hypothalamo–pituitary–adrenal axis." *Frontiers in Neuroendocrinology* 35 (2):197–220. doi: 10.1016/j.yfrne.2013.11.001.

Herrera, Alexandra Ycaza, Howard N. Hodis, Wendy J. Mack, and Mara Mather. 2017. "Estradiol therapy after menopause mitigates effects of stress on cortisol and working memory." *Journal of Clinical Endocrinology & Metabolism* 102 (12):4457–66. doi: 10.1210/jc.2017-00825.

Koch, Patricia Barthalow, Phyllis Kernoff Mansfield, Debra Thurau, and Molly Carey. 2005. "'Feeling frumpy': The relationships between body image and sexual response changes in midlife women." *Journal of Sex Research* 42 (3):215–23. doi: 10.1080/00224490509552276.

Mosconi, Lisa, Valentina Berti, Jonathan Dyke, Eva Schelbaum, Steven Jett, Lacey Loughlin, et al. 2021. "Menopause impacts human brain structure, connectivity, energy metabolism, and amyloid-beta deposition." *Scientific Reports* 11 (1). doi: 10.1038/s41598-021-90084-y.

Ochsner, Kevin N., Jennifer A. Silvers, and Jason T. Buhle. 2012. "Functional imaging studies of emotion regulation: a synthetic review and evolving model of the cognitive control of emotion." *Annals of the New York Academy of Sciences* 1251 (1):E1–E24. doi: 10.1111/j.1749-6632.2012.06751.x.

Pariante, Carmine M., and Stafford L. Lightman. 2008. "The HPA axis in major depression: Classical theories and new developments." *Trends in Neurosciences* 31 (9):464–68. doi: 10.1016/j.tins.2008.06.006.

Parker, Kyle E., Christian E. Pedersen, Adrian M. Gomez, Skylar M. Spangler, Marie C. Walicki, Shelley Y. Feng, et al. 2019. "A paranigral VTA nociceptin circuit that constrains motivation for reward." *Cell* 178 (3):653–71.e19. doi: 10.1016/j.cell.2019.06.034.

Protsenko, Ekaterina, Ruoting Yang, Brent Nier, Victor Reus, Rasha Hammamieh, Ryan Rampersaud, et al. 2021. "'GrimAge,' an epigenetic predictor of mortality, is accelerated in major depressive disorder." *Translational Psychiatry* 11 (1). doi: 10.1038/s41398-021-01302-0.

Sapolsky, Robert M. 2000. "Glucocorticoids and hippocampal atrophy in neuropsychiatric disorders." *Archives of General Psychiatry* 57 (10). doi: 10.1001/archpsyc.57.10.925.

Sherwin, Barbara B. 2012. "Estrogen and cognitive functioning in women: Lessons we have learned." *Behavioral Neuroscience* 126 (1):123–27. doi: 10.1037/a0025539.

Woods, Nancy F., Molly C. Carr, Eunice Y. Tao, Heather J. Taylor, and Ellen S. Mitchell. 2006. "Increased urinary cortisol levels during the menopause transition." *Menopause* 13 (2):212–21. doi: 10.1097/01.gme.0000198490.57242.2e.

Zaki, Jamil, Joshua Ian Davis, and Kevin N. Ochsner. 2012. "Overlapping activity in anterior insula during interoception and emotional experience." *NeuroImage* 62 (1):493–99. doi: 10.1016/j.neuroimage.2012.05.012.

Chapter 6: The Neuroscience of Self-Care

Allen, Andrew P., Timothy G. Dinan, Gerard Clarke, and John F. Cryan. 2017. "A psychology of the human brain-gut-microbiome axis." *Social and Personality Psychology Compass* 11 (4). doi: 10.1111/spc3.12309.

Baer, R. A., J. Carmody, and M. Hunsinger. 2012. "Weekly change in mindfulness and perceived stress in a mindfulness-based stress reduction program." *Journal of Clinical Psychology* 68 (7):755–65. doi: 10.1002/jclp.21865.

Bancos, Simona, Matthew P. Bernard, David J. Topham, and Richard P. Phipps. 2009. "Ibuprofen and other widely used non-steroidal anti-inflammatory drugs inhibit antibody production in human cells." *Cellular Immunology* 258 (1):18–28. doi: 10.1016/j.cellimm.2009.03.007.

Besedovsky, Luciana, Tanja Lange, and Monika Haack. 2019. "The sleep-immune crosstalk in health and disease." *Physiological Reviews* 99 (3):1325–80. doi: 10.1152/physrev.00010.2018.

Boehme, Marcus, Marcel van de Wouw, Thomaz F. S. Bastiaanssen, Loreto Olavarría-Ramírez, Katriona Lyons, Fiona Fouhy, et al. 2019. "Mid-life microbiota crises: Middle age is associated with pervasive neuroimmune alterations that are reversed by targeting the gut microbiome." *Molecular Psychiatry* 25 (10):2567–83. doi: 10.1038/s41380-019-0425-1.

Bonaz, Bruno, Thomas Bazin, and Sonia Pellissier. 2018. "The vagus nerve at the interface of the microbiota-gut-brain axis." *Frontiers in Neuroscience* 12. doi: 10.3389/fnins.2018.00049.

Braun, Theodore P., Xinxia Zhu, Marek Szumowski, Gregory D. Scott, Aaron J. Grossberg, Peter R. Levasseur, et al. 2011. "Central nervous system inflammation induces muscle atrophy via activation of the hypothalamic-pituitary-adrenal axis." *Journal of Experimental Medicine* 208 (12):2449–63. doi: 10.1084/jem.20111020.

Breit, Sigrid, Aleksandra Kupferberg, Gerhard Rogler, and Gregor Hasler. 2018. "Vagus nerve as modulator of the brain-gut axis in psychiatric and inflammatory disorders." *Frontiers in Psychiatry* 9. doi: 10.3389/fpsyt.2018.00044.

Brunt, V. E., R. A. Gioscia-Ryan, J. J. Richey, M. C. Zigler, L. M. Cuevas, A. Gonzalez, et al. 2019. "Suppression of the gut microbiome ameliorates age-related arterial dysfunction and oxidative stress in mice." *Journal of Physiology* 597 (9):2361–78. doi: 10.1113/JP277336.

Burokas, Aurelijus, Silvia Arboleya, Rachel D. Moloney, Veronica L. Peterson, Kiera Murphy, Gerard Clarke, et al. 2017. "Targeting the microbiota-gut-brain axis: Prebiotics have anxiolytic and antidepressant-like effects and reverse the impact of chronic stress in mice." *Biological Psychiatry* 82 (7):472–87. doi: 10.1016/j.biopsych.2016.12.031.

Bussian, T. J., A. Aziz, C. F. Meyer, B. L. Swenson, J. M. van Deursen, and D. J. Baker. 2018. "Clearance of senescent glial cells prevents tau-dependent pathology and cognitive decline." *Nature* 562 (7728):578–82. doi: 10.1038/s41586-018-0543-y.

Cai, Dongsheng, and Sinan Kohr. 2019. "'Hypothalamic microinflammation' paradigm in aging and metabolic diseases." *Cell Metabolism* 30 (1):19–35. doi:10.1016/j.cmet.2019.05.021.

Casaletto, Kaitlin B., Fanny M. Elahi, Adam M. Staffaroni, Samantha Walters, Wilfredo Rivera Contreras, Amy Wolf, et al. 2019. "Cognitive aging is not created

equally: Differentiating unique cognitive phenotypes in 'normal' adults."
Neurobiology of Aging 77:13–19. doi: 10.1016/j.neurobiolaging.2019.01.007.

Collins, F. L., N. D. Rios-Arce, S. Atkinson, H. Bierhalter, D. Schoenherr, J. N.
Bazil, et al. 2017. "Temporal and regional intestinal changes in permeability, tight
junction, and cytokine gene expression following ovariectomy-induced estrogen
deficiency." *Physiological Reports* 5 (9). doi: 10.14814/phy2.13263.

Cryan, John F., Kenneth J. O'Riordan, Kiran Sandhu, Veronica Peterson, and
Timothy G. Dinan. 2020. "The gut microbiome in neurological disorders." *Lancet
Neurology* 19 (2):179–94. doi: 10.1016/s1474-4422(19)30356-4.

Daghlas, Iyas, Jacqueline M. Lane, Richa Saxena, and Céline Vetter. 2021.
"Genetically proxied diurnal preference, sleep timing, and risk of major depressive
disorder." *JAMA Psychiatry* 78 (8):903–10. doi: 10.1001/jamapsychiatry.2021.0959.

Dantzer, Robert. 2018. "Neuroimmune interactions: From the brain to the immune
system and vice versa." *Physiological Reviews* 98 (1):477–504. doi: 10.1152/
physrev.00039.2016.

D'Mello, C., N. Ronaghan, R. Zaheer, M. Dicay, T. Le, W. K. MacNaughton, M. G.
Surrette, and M. G. Swain. 2015. "Probiotics improve inflammation-associated
sickness behavior by altering communication between the peripheral immune
system and the brain." *Journal of Neuroscience* 35 (30):10821–30. doi: 10.1523/
jneurosci.0575-15.2015.

Erickson, Michelle A., William A. Banks, and Robert Dantzer. 2018.
"Neuroimmune axes of the blood-brain barriers and blood-brain interfaces: Bases
for physiological regulation, disease states, and pharmacological interventions."
Pharmacological Reviews 70 (2):278–314. doi: 10.1124/pr.117.014647.

Evrensel, A., B. Onen Unsalver, and M. E. Ceylan. 2019. "Therapeutic potential of
the microbiome in the treatment of neuropsychiatric disorders." *Medical Sciences
(Basel)* 7 (2):21. doi: 10.3390/medsci7020021.

Felger, Jennifer C. 2018. "Imaging the role of inflammation in mood and anxiety-
related disorders." *Current Neuropharmacology* 16 (5):533–58. doi: 10.2174/157015
9x15666171123201142.

Felger, Jennifer C., and Michael T. Treadway. 2016. "Inflammation effects on
motivation and motor activity: role of dopamine." *Neuropsychopharmacology* 42
(1):216–41. doi: 10.1038/npp.2016.143.

Fuhrman, B. J., H. S. Feigelson, R. Flores, M. H. Gail, X. Xu, J. Ravel, and James J.
Goedert. 2014. "Associations of the fecal microbiome with urinary estrogens and
estrogen metabolites in postmenopausal women." *Journal of Clinical Endocrinology
and Metabolism* 99 (12):4632–40. doi: 10.1210/jc.2014-2222.

Fung, T. C., H. E. Vuong, C. D. G. Luna, G. N. Pronovost, A. A. Aleksandrova,
N. G. Riley, et al. 2019. "Intestinal serotonin and fluoxetine exposure modulate

bacterial colonization in the gut." *Nature Microbiology* 4 (12):2064–73. doi: 10.1038/s41564-019-0540-4.

Gibson, Glenn R., Robert Hutkins, Mary Ellen Sanders, Susan L. Prescott, Raylene A. Reimer, Seppo J. Salminen, et al. 2017. "Expert consensus document: The International Scientific Association for Probiotics and Prebiotics (ISAPP) consensus statement on the definition and scope of prebiotics." *Nature Reviews Gastroenterology & Hepatology* 14 (8):491–502. doi: 10.1038/nrgastro.2017.75.

Goverse, Gera, Michelle Stakenborg, and Gianluca Matteoli. 2016. "The intestinal cholinergic anti-inflammatory pathway." *Journal of Physiology* 594 (20):5771–80. doi: 10.1113/jp271537.

Greenfield, Shelly F., Sudie E. Back, Katie Lawson, and Kathleen T. Brady. 2010. "Substance abuse in women." *Psychiatric Clinics of North America* 33 (2):339–55. doi: 10.1016/j.psc.2010.01.004.

Griswold, Max G., Nancy Fullman, Caitlin Hawley, Nicholas Arian, Stephanie R. M. Zimsen, Hayley D. Tymeson, et al. 2018. "Alcohol use and burden for 195 countries and territories, 1990–2016: A systematic analysis for the Global Burden of Disease Study 2016." *Lancet* 392 (10152):1015–35. doi: 10.1016/s0140-6736(18)31310-2.

Harand, Caroline, Françoise Bertran, Franck Doidy, Fabian Guénolé, Béatrice Desgranges, Francis Eustache, and Géraldine Rauchs. 2012. "How aging affects sleep-dependent memory consolidation?" *Frontiers in Neurology* 3. doi: 10.3389/fneur.2012.00008.

Hardeland, Rüdiger. 2019. "Aging, melatonin, and the pro- and anti-inflammatory networks." *International Journal of Molecular Sciences* 20 (5). doi: 10.3390/ijms20051223.

Harper, C. 2009. "The neuropathology of alcohol-related brain damage." *Alcohol and Alcoholism* 44 (2):136–40. doi: 10.1093/alcalc/agn102.

Hilderbrand, Elisa R., and Amy W. Lasek. 2018. "Estradiol enhances ethanol reward in female mice through activation of ERα and ERβ." *Hormones and Behavior* 98:159–64. doi: 10.1016/j.yhbeh.2018.01.001.

Kim, Jee Wook, Dong Young Lee, Boung Chul Lee, Myung Hun Jung, Hano Kim, Yong Sung Choi, and Ihn-Geun Choi. 2012. "Alcohol and cognition in the elderly: A review." *Psychiatry Investigation* 9 (1). doi: 10.4306/pi.2012.9.1.8.

Kim, Sangjune, Seung-Hwan Kwon, Tae-In Kam, Nikhil Panicker, Senthilkumar S. Karuppagounder, Saebom Lee, et al. 2019. "Transneuronal propagation of pathologic α-synuclein from the gut to the brain models Parkinson's disease." *Neuron* 103 (4):627–41.e7. doi: 10.1016/j.neuron.2019.05.035.

Kowalski, K., and A. Mulak. 2019. "Brain-gut-microbiota axis in Alzheimer's disease." *Journal of Neurogastroenterology and Motility* 25 (1):48–60. doi: 10.5056/jnm18087.

Küffer, Andreas, Laura D. Straus, Aric A. Prather, Sabra S. Inslicht, Anne Richards, Judy K. Shigenaga, et al. 2019. "Altered overnight levels of pro-inflammatory cytokines in men and women with posttraumatic stress disorder." *Psychoneuroendocrinology* 102:114–20. doi: 10.1016/j.psyneuen.2018.12.002.

Lindbergh, Cutter A., Kaitlin B. Casaletto, Adam M. Staffaroni, Fanny Elahi, Samantha M. Walters, Michelle You, et al. 2020. "Systemic tumor necrosis factor-alpha trajectories relate to brain health in typically aging older adults." *Journals of Gerontology: Series A* 75 (8):1558–65. doi: 10.1093/gerona/glz209.

Lionnet, Arthur, Laurène Leclair-Visonneau, Michel Neunlist, Shigeo Murayama, Masaki Takao, Charles H. Adler, et al. 2017. "Does Parkinson's disease start in the gut?" *Acta Neuropathologica* 135 (1):1–12. doi: 10.1007/s00401-017-1777-8.

Liu, Jing, Fei Xu, Zhiyan Nie, and Lei Shao. 2020. "Gut microbiota approach—a new strategy to treat Parkinson's disease." *Frontiers in Cellular and Infection Microbiology* 10. doi: 10.3389/fcimb.2020.570658.

Lobionda, Stefani, Panida Sittipo, Hyog Young Kwon, and Yun Kyung Lee. 2019. "The role of gut microbiota in intestinal inflammation with respect to diet and extrinsic stressors." *Microorganisms* 7 (8). doi: 10.3390/microorganisms7080271.

Martin, Dominique E., Blake L. Torrance, Laura Haynes, and Jenna M. Bartley. 2021. "Targeting aging: Lessons learned from immunometabolism and cellular senescence." *Frontiers in Immunology* 12. doi: 10.3389/fimmu.2021.714742.

Michaud, Martin, Laurent Balardy, Guillaume Moulis, Clement Gaudin, Caroline Peyrot, Bruno Vellas, et al. 2013. "Proinflammatory cytokines, aging, and age-related diseases." *Journal of the American Medical Directors Association* 14 (12):877–82. doi: 10.1016/j.jamda.2013.05.009.

Miller, Andrew H., Ebrahim Haroon, Charles L. Raison, and Jennifer C. Felger. 2013. "Cytokine targets in the brain: Impact on neurotransmitters and neurocircuits." *Depression and Anxiety* 30 (4):297–306. doi: 10.1002/da.22084.

Milton, David C., Joey Ward, Emilia Ward, Donald M. Lyall, Rona J. Strawbridge, Daniel J. Smith, and Breda Cullen. 2021. "The association between C-reactive protein, mood disorder, and cognitive function in UK Biobank." *European Psychiatry* 64 (1). doi: 10.1192/j.eurpsy.2021.6.

Moieni, Mona, Kevin M. Tan, Tristen K. Inagaki, Keely A. Muscatell, Janine M. Dutcher, Ivana Jevtic, et al. 2019. "Sex differences in the relationship between inflammation and reward sensitivity: A randomized controlled trial of endotoxin." *Biological Psychiatry: Cognitive Neuroscience and Neuroimaging* 4 (7):619–26. doi: 10.1016/j.bpsc.2019.03.010.

Mu, Qinghui, Vincent J. Tavella, and Xin M. Luo. 2018. "Role of *Lactobacillus reuteri* in human health and diseases." *Frontiers in Microbiology* 9. doi: 10.3389/fmicb.2018.00757.

Mursu, Jaakko, Lyn M. Steffen, Katie A. Meyer, Daniel Duprez, and David R. Jacobs. 2013. "Diet quality indexes and mortality in postmenopausal women: The Iowa Women's Health Study." *American Journal of Clinical Nutrition* 98 (2):444–53. doi: 10.3945/ajcn.112.055681.

Niles, Andrea N., Mariya Smirnova, Joy Lin, and Aoife O'Donovan. 2018. "Gender differences in longitudinal relationships between depression and anxiety symptoms and inflammation in the health and retirement study." *Psychoneuroendocrinology* 95:149–57. doi: 10.1016/j.psyneuen.2018.05.035.

Oslin, David W., and Mark S. Cary. 2003. "Alcohol-related dementia: Validation of diagnostic criteria." *American Journal of Geriatric Psychiatry* 11 (4):441–47. doi: 10.1097/00019442-200307000-00007.

Pace, Thaddeus W. W., Lobsang Tenzin Negi, Daniel D. Adame, Steven P. Cole, Teresa I. Sivilli, Timothy D. Brown, et al. 2009. "Effect of compassion meditation on neuroendocrine, innate immune and behavioral responses to psychosocial stress." *Psychoneuroendocrinology* 34 (1):87–98. doi: 10.1016/j.psyneuen.2008.08.011.

Peterson, Christine Tara. 2020. "Dysfunction of the microbiota-gut-brain axis in neurodegenerative disease: The promise of therapeutic modulation with prebiotics, medicinal herbs, probiotics, and synbiotics." *Journal of Evidence-Based Integrative Medicine* 25 (1). doi: 10.1177/2515690x20957225.

Polloni, Laura, and Antonella Muraro. 2020. "Anxiety and food allergy: A review of the last two decades." *Clinical & Experimental Allergy* 50 (4):420–41. doi: 10.1111/cea.13548.

Rehm, Jürgen, Omer S. M. Hasan, Sandra E. Black, Kevin D. Shield, and Michaël Schwarzinger. 2019. "Alcohol use and dementia: A systematic scoping review." *Alzheimer's Research & Therapy* 11 (1). doi: 10.1186/s13195-018-0453-0.

Ridley, Nicole J., Brian Draper, and Adrienne Withall. 2013. "Alcohol-related dementia: An update of the evidence." *Alzheimer's Research & Therapy* 5 (1). doi: 10.1186/alzrt157.

Sayed, Nazish, Yingxiang Huang, Khiem Nguyen, Zuzana Krejciova-Rajaniemi, Anissa P. Grawe, Tianxiang Gao, et al. 2021. "An inflammatory aging clock (iAge) based on deep learning tracks multimorbidity, immunosenescence, frailty and cardiovascular aging." *Nature Aging* 1 (7):598–615. doi: 10.1038/s43587-021-00082-y.

Schiffrin, E. J., D. R. Thomas, V. B. Kumar, C. Brown, C. Hager, M. A. Van't Hof, et al. 2007. "Systemic inflammatory markers in older persons: the effect of oral nutritional supplementation with prebiotics." *Journal of Nutrition, Health & Aging* 11 (6):475–79.

Sovijit, Watcharin N., Watcharee E. Sovijit, Shaoxia Pu, Kento Usuda, Ryo Inoue, Gen Watanabe, et al. 2021. "Ovarian progesterone suppresses depression and anxiety-like behaviors by increasing the Lactobacillus population of gut microbiota in ovariectomized mice." *Neuroscience Research* 168:76–82. doi: 10.1016/j.neures.2019.04.005.

Sohn, Emily. 2021. "Why autoimmunity is most common in women." *Nature* 595 (7867):S51–S53. doi: 10.1038/d41586-021-01836-9.

Ticinesi, Andrea, Claudio Tana, Antonio Nouvenne, Beatrice Prati, Fulvio Lauretani, and Tiziana Meschi. 2018. "Gut microbiota, cognitive frailty and dementia in older individuals: A systematic review." *Clinical Interventions in Aging* 13:1497–511. doi: 10.2147/cia.S139163.

Van Houten, J. M., R. J. Wessells, H. L. Lujan, and S. E. DiCarlo. 2015. "My gut feeling says rest: Increased intestinal permeability contributes to chronic diseases in high-intensity exercisers." *Medical Hypotheses* 85 (6):882–86. doi: 10.1016/j.mehy.2015.09.018.

Vieira, Angélica T., Paula M. Castelo, Daniel A. Ribeiro, and Caroline M. Ferreira. 2017. "Influence of oral and gut microbiota in the health of menopausal women." *Frontiers in Microbiology* 8. doi: 10.3389/fmicb.2017.01884.

Vulevic, Jelena, Alexandra Drakoularakou, Parveen Yaqoob, George Tzortzis, and Glenn R. Gibson. 2008. "Modulation of the fecal microflora profile and immune function by a novel trans-galactooligosaccharide mixture (B-GOS) in healthy elderly volunteers." *American Journal of Clinical Nutrition* 88 (5):1438–46. doi: 10.3945/ajcn.2008.26242.

Walker, Keenan A., Ron C. Hoogeveen, Aaron R. Folsom, Christie M. Ballantyne, David S. Knopman, B. Gwen Windham, et al. 2017. "Midlife systemic inflammatory markers are associated with late-life brain volume." *Neurology* 89 (22):2262–70. doi: 10.1212/wnl.0000000000004688.

Xie, Ruining, Pei Jiang, Li Lin, Jian Jiang, Bin Yu, Jingjing Rao, et al. 2020. "Oral treatment with *Lactobacillus reuteri* attenuates depressive-like behaviors and serotonin metabolism alterations induced by chronic social defeat stress." *Journal of Psychiatric Research* 122:70–78. doi: 10.1016/j.jpsychires.2019.12.013.

Xu, Ming, Tamar Pirtskhalava, Joshua N. Farr, Bettina M. Weigand, Allyson K. Palmer, Megan M. Weivoda, et al. 2018. "Senolytics improve physical function and increase lifespan in old age." *Nature Medicine* 24 (8):1246–56. doi: 10.1038/s41591-018-0092-9.

Yoon, Kichul, and Nayoung Kim. 2021. "Roles of sex hormones and gender in the gut microbiota." *Journal of Neurogastroenterology and Motility* 27 (3):314–25. doi: 10.5056/jnm20208.

Zahr, N. M., and A. Pfefferbaum. 2017. "Alcohol's effects on the brain: Neuroimaging results in humans and animal models." *Alcohol Research* 38 (2):183–206.

Chapter 7: Your Brain in Search of Connection

Cacioppo, John T., and William Patrick. *Loneliness: Human Nature and the Need for Social Connection*. New York: W. W. Norton, 2009.

Dölen, Gül, and Robert C. Malenka. 2014. "The emerging role of nucleus accumbens oxytocin in social cognition." *Biological Psychiatry* 76 (5):354–55. doi: 10.1016/j.biopsych.2014.06.009.

Eisenberger, Naomi I., and Matthew D. Lieberman. 2004. "Why rejection hurts: A common neural alarm system for physical and social pain." *Trends in Cognitive Sciences* 8 (7):294–300. doi: 10.1016/j.tics.2004.05.010.

Holt-Lunstad, J., T. B. Smith, M. Baker, T. Harris, and D. Stephenson. 2015. "Loneliness and social isolation as risk factors for mortality: A meta-analytic review." *Perspectives on Psychological Science* 10 (2):227–37. doi: 10.1177/1745691614568352.

Jiang, Luo-Luo, Tamas David-Barrett, Anna Rotkirch, James Carney, Isabel Behncke Izquierdo, Jaimie A. Krems, et al. 2015. "Women favour dyadic relationships, but men prefer clubs: Cross-cultural evidence from social networking." *PLOS ONE* 10 (3). doi: 10.1371/journal.pone.0118329.

Kaufman, Scott B. 2019. "Taking Sex Differences in Personality Seriously." *Scientific American*.

Kudwa, Andrea E., Robert F. McGivern, and Robert J. Handa. 2014. "Estrogen receptor β and oxytocin interact to modulate anxiety-like behavior and neuroendocrine stress reactivity in adult male and female rats." *Physiology & Behavior* 129:287–96. doi: 10.1016/j.physbeh.2014.03.004.

Laakasuo, Michael, Anna Rotkirch, Max van Duijn, Venla Berg, Markus Jokela, Tamas David-Barrett, et al. 2020. "Homophily in personality enhances group success among real-life friends." *Frontiers in Psychology* 11. doi: 10.3389/fpsyg.2020.00710.

Luo, Ye, Louise C. Hawkley, Linda J. Waite, and John T. Cacioppo. 2012. "Loneliness, health, and mortality in old age: A national longitudinal study." *Social Science & Medicine* 74 (6):907–14. doi: 10.1016/j.socscimed.2011.11.028.

Chapter 8: Upgrading the Mommy Brain

Isay, Jane. *Walking on Eggshells: Navigating the Delicate Relationship Between Adult Children and Their Parents*. New York: Broadway Books/Flying Dolphin Press, 2008.

Li, Tong, Ping Wang, Stephani C. Wang, and Yu-Feng Wang. 2017. "Approaches mediating oxytocin regulation of the immune system." *Frontiers in Immunology* 7. doi: 10.3389/fimmu.2016.00693.

Wirth, Michelle M. 2014. "Hormones, stress, and cognition: The effects of glucocorticoids and oxytocin on memory." *Adaptive Human Behavior and Physiology* 1 (2):177–201. doi: 10.1007/s40750-014-0010-4.

Chapter 9: The Relationship Brain

Caldwell, Heather K., and H. Elliott Albers. 2016. "Oxytocin, vasopressin, and the motivational forces that drive social behaviors." *Current Topics in Behavioral Neurosciences* 27:51–103. doi: 10.1007/7854_2015_390.

Dumais, Kelly M., and Alexa H. Veenema. 2016. "Vasopressin and oxytocin receptor systems in the brain: Sex differences and sex-specific regulation of social behavior." *Frontiers in Neuroendocrinology* 40:1–23. doi: 10.1016/j.yfrne.2015.04.003.

Huang, M., S. Su, J. Goldberg, A. H. Miller, O. M. Levantsevych, L. Shallenberger, et al. 2019. "Longitudinal association of inflammation with depressive symptoms: A 7-year cross-lagged twin difference study." *Brain, Behavior, and Immunity* 75:200–207. doi: 10.1016/j.bbi.2018.10.007.

Langer, Ellen J. *Mindfulness.* Massachusetts: Addison-Wesley, 1989.

Maffei, L., E. Picano, M. G. Andreassi, A. Angelucci, F Baldacci, L. Baroncelli, et al. 2017. "Randomized trial on the effects of a combined physical/cognitive training in aged MCI subjects: The Train the Brain study." *Scientific Reports* 7 (1). doi: 10.1038/srep39471.

Niles, A. N., M. Smirnova, J. Lin, and A. O'Donovan. 2018. "Gender differences in longitudinal relationships between depression and anxiety symptoms and inflammation in the health and retirement study." *Psychoneuroendocrinology* 95:149–57. doi: 10.1016/j.psyneuen.2018.05.035.

Sharma, Animesh N., Paul Aoun, Jean R. Wigham, Suanne M. Weist, and Johannes D. Veldhuis. 2014. "Estradiol, but not testosterone, heightens cortisol-mediated negative feedback on pulsatile ACTH secretion and ACTH approximate entropy in unstressed older men and women." *American Journal of Physiology-Regulatory, Integrative and Comparative Physiology* 306 (9):R627–35. doi: 10.1152/ajpregu.00551.2013.

Shrout, M. Rosie, Randal D. Brown, Terri L. Orbuch, and Daniel J. Weigel. 2019. "A multidimensional examination of marital conflict and subjective health over 16 years." *Personal Relationships* 26 (3):490–506. doi: 10.1111/pere.12292.

Smith, B. M., X. Yao, K. S. Chen, and E. D. Kirby. 2018. "A larger social network enhances novel object location memory and reduces hippocampal microgliosis in aged mice." *Frontiers in Aging Neuroscience* 10:142. doi: 10.3389/fnagi.2018.00142.

Chapter 10: Centering

Boyle, Christina P., Cyrus A. Raji, Kirk I. Erickson, Oscar L. Lopez, James T. Becker, H. Michael Gach, et al. 2020. "Estrogen, brain structure, and cognition in postmenopausal women." *Human Brain Mapping* 42 (1):24–35. doi: 10.1002/hbm.25200.

Uddin, Lucina Q. 2014. "Salience processing and insular cortical function and dysfunction." *Nature Reviews Neuroscience* 16 (1):55–61. doi: 10.1038/nrn3857.

Chapter 11: Body Hacks for the Mind

Adamaszek, M., F. D'Agata, R. Ferrucci, C. Habas, S. Keulen, K. C. Kirkby, et al. 2016. "Consensus paper: Cerebellum and emotion." *Cerebellum* 16 (2):552–76. doi: 10.1007/s12311-016-0815-8.

Bloss, E. B., W. G. Janssen, B. S. McEwen, and J. H. Morrison. 2010. "Interactive effects of stress and aging on structural plasticity in the prefrontal cortex." *Journal of Neuroscience* 30 (19):6726–31. doi: 10.1523/jneurosci.0759-10.2010.

Borhan, A. S. M., Patricia Hewston, Dafna Merom, Courtney Kennedy, George Ioannidis, Nancy Santesso, et al. 2018. "Effects of dance on cognitive function among older adults: A protocol for systematic review and meta-analysis." *Systematic Reviews* 7 (1). doi: 10.1186/s13643-018-0689-6.

Brown, Stuart L., and Christopher C. Vaughan. *Play: How It Shapes the Brain, Opens the Imagination, and Invigorates the Soul.* New York: Avery, 2010.

Casaletto, Kaitlin B., Adam M. Staffaroni, Fanny Elahi, Emily Fox, Persephone A. Crittenden, Michelle You, et al. 2018. "Perceived stress is associated with accelerated Monocyte/Macrophage aging trajectories in clinically normal adults." *American Journal of Geriatric Psychiatry* 26 (9):952–63. doi: 10.1016/j.jagp.2018.05.004.

D'Angelo, Egidio. 2019. "The cerebellum gets social." *Science* 363 (6424):229. doi: 10.1126/science.aaw2571.

de Kloet, E. Ron, Marian Joëls, and Florian Holsboer. 2005. "Stress and the brain: From adaptation to disease." *Nature Reviews Neuroscience* 6 (6):463–75. doi: 10.1038/nrn1683.

de Oliveira Matos, Felipe, Amanda Vido, William Fernando Garcia, Wendell Arthur Lopes, and Antonio Pereira. 2020. "A neurovisceral integrative study on cognition, heart rate variability, and fitness in the elderly." *Frontiers in Aging Neuroscience* 12. doi: 10.3389/fnagi.2020.00051.

Devita, Maria, Francesco Alberti, Michela Fagnani, Fabio Masina, Enrica Ara, Giuseppe Sergi, et al. 2021. "Novel insights into the relationship between cerebellum and dementia: A narrative review as a toolkit for clinicians." *Ageing Research Reviews* 70. doi: 10.1016/j.arr.2021.101389.

Ding, Kan, Takashi Tarumi, David C. Zhu, Benjamin Y. Tseng, Binu P. Thomas, Marcel Turner, et al. 2017. "Cardiorespiratory fitness and white matter neuronal fiber integrity in mild cognitive impairment." *Journal of Alzheimer's Disease* 61 (2):729–39. doi: 10.3233/jad-170415.

Erickson, K. I., M. W. Voss, R. S. Prakash, C. Basak, A. Szabo, L. Chaddock, et al. 2011. "Exercise training increases size of hippocampus and improves memory." *Proceedings of the National Academy of Sciences* 108 (7):3017–22. doi: 10.1073/pnas.1015950108.

Killingsworth, M. A., Gilbert, D. T., 2010 "A wandering mind is an unhappy mind." *Science,* 330 (6006):932. doi: 10.1126/science.1192439.

Lavretsky, Helen, and Paul A. Newhouse. 2012. "Stress, inflammation, and aging." *American Journal of Geriatric Psychiatry* 20 (9):729–33. doi: 10.1097/JGP.0b013e31826573cf.

Leggio, Maria, and Giusy Olivito. 2018. "Topography of the cerebellum in relation to social brain regions and emotions." *Handbook of Clinical Neurology* 154:71–84. doi: 10.1016/B978-0-444-63956-1.

Marek, Scott, Joshua S. Siegel, Evan M. Gordon, Ryan V. Raut, Caterina Gratton, Dillan J. Newbold, et al. 2018. "Spatial and temporal organization of the individual human cerebellum." *Neuron* 100 (4):977–93.e7. doi: 10.1016/j.neuron.2018.10.010.

Matyi, Joshua M., Gail B. Rattinger, Sarah Schwartz, Mona Buhusi, and JoAnn T. Tschanz. 2019. "Lifetime estrogen exposure and cognition in late life: The Cache County Study." *Menopause* 26 (12):1366–74. doi: 10.1097/gme.0000000000001405.

McEwen, Bruce S. 2019. "What is the confusion with cortisol?" *Chronic Stress* 3. doi: 10.1177/2470547019833647.

Mishra, Aarti, Yuan Shang, Yiwei Wang, Eliza R. Bacon, Fei Yin, and Roberta D. Brinton. 2020. "Dynamic neuroimmune profile during mid-life aging in the female brain and implications for Alzheimer risk." *iScience* 23 (12). doi: 10.1016/j.isci.2020.101829.

Murri, Martino Belvederi, Federico Triolo, Alice Coni, Carlo Tacconi, Erika Nerozzi, Andrea Escelsior, et al. 2020. "Instrumental assessment of balance and gait in depression: A systematic review." *Psychiatry Research* 284. doi: 10.1016/j.psychres.2019.112687.

Ochs-Balcom, Heather M., Leah Preus, Jing Nie, Jean Wactawski-Wende, Linda Agyemang, Marian L. Neuhouser, et al. 2018. "Physical activity modifies genetic susceptibility to obesity in postmenopausal women." *Menopause* 25 (10):1131–37. doi: 10.1097/gme.0000000000001134.

Schmahmann, Jeremy D. 2019. "The cerebellum and cognition." *Neuroscience Letters* 688:62–75. doi: 10.1016/j.neulet.2018.07.005.

Shrout, M. Rosie, Megan E. Renna, Annelise A. Madison, Lisa M. Jaremka, Christopher P. Fagundes, William B. Malarkey, and Janice Kiecolt-Glaser. 2020. "Cortisol slopes and conflict: A spouse's perceived stress matters." *Psychoneuroendocrinology* 121. doi: 10.1016/j.psyneuen.2020.104839.

Siviy, Stephen M. 2016. "A brain motivated to play: Insights into the neurobiology of playfulness." *Behaviour* 153 (6–7):819–44. doi: 10.1163/1568539x-00003349.

Söderkvist, Sven, Kajsa Ohlén, and Ulf Dimberg. 2017. "How the experience of emotion is modulated by facial feedback." *Journal of Nonverbal Behavior* 42 (1):129–51. doi: 10.1007/s10919-017-0264-1.

Strata, Piergiorgio. 2015. "The emotional cerebellum." *Cerebellum* 14 (5):570–77. doi: 10.1007/s12311-015-0649-9.

Topp, Robert, Marcia Ditmyer, Karen King, Kristen Doherty, and Joseph Hornyak. 2002. "The effect of bed rest and potential of prehabilitation on patients in the intensive care unit." *AACN Clinical Issues: Advanced Practice in Acute and Critical Care* 13 (2):263–76. doi: 10.1097/00044067-200205000-00011.

Traustadóttir, Tinna, Pamela R. Bosch, and Kathleen S. Matt. 2005. "The HPA axis response to stress in women: Effects of aging and fitness." *Psychoneuroendocrinology* 30 (4):392–402. doi: 10.1016/j.psyneuen.2004.11.002.

Vecchio, Laura M., Ying Meng, Kristiana Xhima, Nir Lipsman, Clement Hamani, Isabelle Aubert, et al. 2018. "The neuroprotective effects of exercise: Maintaining a healthy brain throughout aging." *Brain Plasticity* 4 (1):17–52. doi: 10.3233/bpl-180069.

Weitz, Gunther, Mikael Elam, Jan Born, Horst L. Fehm, and Christoph Dodt. 2001. "Postmenopausal estrogen administration suppresses muscle sympathetic nerve activity." *Journal of Clinical Endocrinology & Metabolism* 86 (1):344–48. doi: 10.1210/jcem.86.1.7138.

Chapter 12: The Return of Purpose

Baune, Bernhard, Antoine Lutz, Julie Brefczynski-Lewis, Tom Johnstone, and Richard J. Davidson. 2008. "Regulation of the neural circuitry of emotion by compassion meditation: Effects of meditative expertise." *PLOS ONE* 3 (3). doi: 10.1371/journal.pone.0001897.

Hedegaard, Holly, Sally C. Curtin, and Margaret Warner. "Suicide mortality in the United States, 1999–2017." NCHS Data Brief No. 330, November 2018.

Litzelman, Kristin, Whitney P. Witt, Ronald E. Gangnon, F. Javier Nieto, Corinne D. Engelman, Marsha R. Mailick, and Halcyon Gerald Skinner. 2014. "Association between informal caregiving and cellular aging in the Survey of the Health of Wisconsin: The role of caregiving characteristics, stress, and strain." *American Journal of Epidemiology* 179 (11):1340–52. doi: 10.1093/aje/kwu066.

López-Otín, Carlos, Maria A. Blasco, Linda Partridge, Manuel Serrano, and Guido Kroemer. 2013. "The hallmarks of aging." *Cell* 153 (6):1194–217. doi: 10.1016/j.cell.2013.05.039.

Chapter 13: New Focus

Al-Hashimi, Omar, Theodore P. Zanto, and Adam Gazzaley. 2015. "Neural sources of performance decline during continuous multitasking." *Cortex* 71:49–57. doi: 10.1016/j.cortex.2015.06.001.

Anguera, J. A., J. Boccanfuso, J. L. Rintoul, O. Al-Hashimi, F. Faraji, J. Janowich, et al. 2013. "Video game training enhances cognitive control in older adults." *Nature* 501 (7465):97–101. doi: 10.1038/nature12486.

Anguera, Joaquin A., Jessica N. Schachtner, Alexander J. Simon, Joshua Volponi, Samirah Javed, Courtney L. Gallen, and Adam Gazzaley. 2021. "Long-term maintenance of multitasking abilities following video game training in older adults." *Neurobiology of Aging* 103:22–30. doi: 10.1016/j.neurobiolaging.2021.02.023.

Bratman, Gregory N., J. Paul Hamilton, Kevin S. Hahn, Gretchen C. Daily, and James J. Gross. 2015. "Nature experience reduces rumination and subgenual prefrontal cortex activation." *Proceedings of the National Academy of Sciences* 112 (28):8567–72. doi: 10.1073/pnas.1510459112.

Clapp, W. C., M. T. Rubens, J. Sabharwal, and A. Gazzaley. 2011. "Deficit in switching between functional brain networks underlies the impact of multitasking on working memory in older adults." *Proceedings of the National Academy of Sciences* 108 (17):7212–17. doi: 10.1073/pnas.1015297108.

Frago, Laura M., Sandra Canelles, Alejandra Freire-Regatillo, Pilar Argente-Arizón, Vicente Barrios, Jesús Argente, et al. 2017. "Estradiol uses different mechanisms in astrocytes from the hippocampus of male and female rats to protect against damage induced by palmitic acid." *Frontiers in Molecular Neuroscience* 10. doi: 10.3389/fnmol.2017.00330.

Kim, Yu Jin, Maira Soto, Gregory L. Branigan, Kathleen Rodgers, and Roberta Diaz Brinton. 2021. "Association between menopausal hormone therapy and risk of neurodegenerative diseases: Implications for precision hormone therapy." *Alzheimer's & Dementia: Translational Research & Clinical Interventions* 7 (1). doi: 10.1002/trc2.12174.

Reuter-Lorenz, Patricia A., and Denise C. Park. 2014. "How does it STAC up? Revisiting the scaffolding theory of aging and cognition." *Neuropsychology Review* 24 (3):355–70. doi: 10.1007/s11065-014-9270-9.

Sherwin, Barbara B. 2008. "Hormones, the brain, and me." *Canadian Psychology/Psychologie canadienne* 49 (1):42–48. doi: 10.1037/0708-5591.49.1.42.

Tsuchiyagaito, Aki, Masaya Misaki, Obada Al Zoubi, Martin Paulus, and Jerzy Bodurka. 2020. "Prevent breaking bad: A proof of concept study of rebalancing the brain's rumination circuit with real-time fMRI functional connectivity neurofeedback." *Human Brain Mapping* 42 (4):922–40. doi: 10.1002/hbm.25268.

Chapter 14: Life Span or Health Span?

Brinton, Roberta Diaz. 2008. "Estrogen regulation of glucose metabolism and mitochondrial function: Therapeutic implications for prevention of Alzheimer's disease." *Advanced Drug Delivery Reviews* 60 (13–14):1504–11. doi: 10.1016/j.addr.2008.06.003.

Chowen, Julie A., and Luis M. Garcia-Segura. 2021. "Role of glial cells in the generation of sex differences in neurodegenerative diseases and brain aging." *Mechanisms of Ageing and Development* 196. doi: 10.1016/j.mad.2021.111473.

Dubal, Dena B. 2020. "Sex difference in Alzheimer's disease: An updated, balanced and emerging perspective on differing vulnerabilities." *Handbook of Clinical Neurology* 175:261–73. doi: 10.1016/B978-0-444-64123-6.00018-7.

Dumas, Julie, Catherine Hancur-Bucci, Magdalena Naylor, Cynthia Sites, and Paul Newhouse. 2008. "Estradiol interacts with the cholinergic system to affect verbal memory in postmenopausal women: Evidence for the critical period hypothesis." *Hormones and Behavior* 53 (1):159–69. doi: 10.1016/j.yhbeh.2007.09.011.

Etnier, Jennifer L., Eric S. Drollette, and Alexis B. Slutsky. 2019. "Physical activity and cognition: A narrative review of the evidence for older adults." *Psychology of Sport and Exercise* 42:156–66. doi: 10.1016/j.psychsport.2018.12.006.

Fassier, Philippine, Jae Hee Kang, I. Min Lee, Francine Grodstein, and Marie-Noël Vercambre. 2021. "Vigorous physical activity and cognitive trajectory later in life: Prospective association and interaction by apolipoprotein E e4 in the Nurses' Health Study." *Journals of Gerontology: Series A*. doi: 10.1093/gerona/glab169.

Fisher, Daniel W., David A. Bennett, and Hongxin Dong. 2018. "Sexual dimorphism in predisposition to Alzheimer's disease." *Neurobiology of Aging* 70:308–24. doi: 10.1016/j.neurobiolaging.2018.04.004.

Grodstein, Francine, Jennifer Chen, Daniel A. Pollen, Marilyn S. Albert, Robert S. Wilson, Marshal F. Folstein, et al. 2000. "Postmenopausal hormone therapy and cognitive function in healthy older women." *Journal of the American Geriatrics Society* 48 (7):746–52. doi: 10.1111/j.1532-5415.2000.tb04748.x.

Jiménez-Balado, Joan, and Teal S. Eich. 2021. "GABAergic dysfunction, neural network hyperactivity and memory impairments in human aging and Alzheimer's disease." *Seminars in Cell & Developmental Biology* 116:146–59. doi: 10.1016/j.semcdb.2021.01.005.

Klosinski, Lauren P., Jia Yao, Fei Yin, Alfred N. Fonteh, Michael G. Harrington, Trace A. Christensen, et al. 2015. "White matter lipids as a ketogenic fuel supply in aging female brain: Implications for Alzheimer's disease." *EBioMedicine* 2 (12):1888–904. doi: 10.1016/j.ebiom.2015.11.002.

Leng, Yue, and Kristine Yaffe. 2020. "Sleep duration and cognitive aging—beyond a U-shaped association." *JAMA Network Open* 3 (9). doi: 10.1001/jamanetworkopen.2020.14008.

Marin, Raquel, and Mario Diaz. 2018. "Estrogen interactions with lipid rafts related to neuroprotection. Impact of brain ageing and menopause." *Frontiers in Neuroscience* 12. doi: 10.3389/fnins.2018.00128.

Mehta, Jaya, Juliana M. Kling, and JoAnn E. Manson. 2021. "Risks, benefits, and treatment modalities of menopausal hormone therapy: Current concepts." *Frontiers in Endocrinology* 12. doi: 10.3389/fendo.2021.564781.

Mulnard, Ruth A., Carl W. Cotman, Claudia Kawas, Christopher H. van Dyck, Mary Sano, Rachelle Doody, et al. 2000. "Estrogen replacement therapy for treatment of mild to moderate Alzheimer disease." *JAMA* 283 (8):1107–15. doi: 10.1001/jama.283.8.1007.

Paganini-Hill, Annlia, Claudia H. Kawas, and Maria M. Corrada. 2016. "Lifestyle factors and dementia in the oldest-old: The 90+ Study." *Alzheimer Disease & Associated Disorders* 30 (1):21–26. doi: 10.1097/wad.0000000000000087.

Shin, Jean, Stephanie Pelletier, Louis Richer, G. Bruce Pike, Daniel Gaudet, Tomas Paus, and Zdenka Pausova. 2020. "Adiposity-related insulin resistance and thickness of the cerebral cortex in middle-aged adults." *Journal of Neuroendocrinology* 32 (12). doi: 10.1111/jne.12921.

Shumaker, Sally A., Claudine Legault, Stephen R. Rapp, Leon Thal, Robert B. Wallace, Judith K. Ockene, et al. 2003. "Estrogen plus progestin and the incidence of dementia and mild cognitive impairment in postmenopausal women." *JAMA* 289 (20): 2651–62. doi: 10.1001/jama.289.20.2651.

Subramaniapillai, Sivaniya, Anne Almey, M. Natasha Rajah, and Gillian Einstein. 2021. "Sex and gender differences in cognitive and brain reserve: Implications for Alzheimer's disease in women." *Frontiers in Neuroendocrinology* 60. doi: 10.1016/j.yfrne.2020.100879.

Thurston, Rebecca C., Howard J. Aizenstein, Carol A. Derby, Ervin Sejdić, and Pauline M. Maki. 2016. "Menopausal hot flashes and white matter hyperintensities." *Menopause* 23 (1):27–32. doi: 10.1097/gme.0000000000000481.

Wang, Dan, Xuan Wang, Meng-Ting Luo, Hui Wang, and Yue-Hua Li. 2019. "Gamma-aminobutyric acid levels in the anterior cingulate cortex of perimenopausal women with depression: A magnetic resonance spectroscopy study." *Frontiers in Neuroscience* 13. doi: 10.3389/fnins.2019.00785.

Watermeyer, Tamlyn, Catherine Robb, Sarah Gregory, and Chinedu Udeh-Momoh. 2021. "Therapeutic implications of hypothalamic-pituitaryadrenal-axis modulation in Alzheimer's disease: A narrative review of pharmacological and lifestyle interventions." *Frontiers in Neuroendocrinology* 60. doi: 10.1016/j.yfrne.2020.100877.

Wingfield, Arthur, and Jonathan E. Peelle. 2012. "How does hearing loss affect the brain?" *Aging Health* 8 (2):107–9. doi: 10.2217/ahe.12.5.

Yaffe, Kristine, Warren Browner, Jane Cauley, Lenore Launer, and Tamara Harris. 1999. "Association between bone mineral density and cognitive decline in older women." *Journal of the American Geriatrics Society* 47 (10):1176–82. doi: 10.1111/j.1532-5415.1999.tb05196.x.

Yaffe, Kristine, Cherie Falvey, Nathan Hamilton, Ann V. Schwartz, Eleanor M. Simonsick, Suzanne Satterfield, et al. 2012. "Diabetes, glucose control, and 9-year cognitive decline among older adults without dementia." *Archives of Neurology* 69 (9):1170–754. doi: 10.1001/archneurol.2012.1117.

Chapter 15: So Many Transitions

Gehlek, Nawang, Gini Alhadeff, and Mark Magill. *Good Life, Good Death: Tibetan Wisdom.* New York: Riverhead Books, 2001.

Kondziella, Daniel. 2020. "The neurology of death and the dying brain: A pictorial essay." *Frontiers in Neurology* 11. doi: 10.3389/fneur.2020.00736.

Parnia, Sam, Tara Keshavarz, Meghan McMullin, and Tori Williams. 2019. "Abstract 387: Awareness and cognitive activity during cardiac arrest." *Circulation* 140 (Suppl_2). doi: 10.1161/circ.140.suppl_2.387.

Rady, Mohamed Y., and Joseph L. Verheijde. 2016. "Neuroscience and awareness in the dying human brain: Implications for organ donation practices." *Journal of Critical Care* 34:121–23. doi: 10.1016/j.jcrc.2016.04.016.

Appendix

American Geriatrics Society 2019. "American Geriatrics Society 2019 updated AGS Beers Criteria® for potentially inappropriate medication use in older adults." *Journal of the American Geriatrics Society* 67 (4):674–94. doi: 10.1111/jgs.15767.

Baum, Jamie, Il-Young Kim, and Robert Wolfe. 2016. "Protein consumption and the elderly: what is the optimal level of intake?" *Nutrients* 8 (6). doi: 10.3390/nu8060359.

Baune, Bernhard, Antoine Lutz, Julie Brefczynski-Lewis, Tom Johnstone, and Richard J. Davidson. 2008. "Regulation of the neural circuitry of emotion by compassion meditation: Effects of meditative expertise." *PLOS ONE* 3 (3). doi: 10.1371/journal.pone.0001897.

Blumenthal, James A., Patrick J. Smith, and Benson M. Hoffman. 2012. "Is exercise a viable treatment for depression?" *ACSM'S Health & Fitness Journal* 16 (4):14–21. doi: 10.1249/01.FIT.0000416000.09526.eb.

Borghesan, M., W. M. H. Hoogaars, M. Varela-Eirin, N. Talma, and M. Demaria. 2020. "A senescence-centric view of aging: Implications for longevity and disease." *Trends in Cell Biology* 30 (10):777–91. doi: 10.1016/j.tcb.2020.07.002.

Buchowski, Maciej S., Kathrin Rehfeld, Angie Lüders, Anita Hökelmann, Volkmar Lessmann, Joern Kaufmann, et al. 2018. "Dance training is superior to repetitive physical exercise in inducing brain plasticity in the elderly." *PLOS ONE* 13 (7). doi: 10.1371/journal.pone.0196636.

Cai, Dongsheng, and Sinan Kohr. 2019. "'Hypothalamic microinflammation' paradigm in aging and metabolic diseases." *Cell Metabolism* 30 (1):19–35. doi: 10.1016/j.cmet.2019.05.021.

Collins, Nicholas, Natalia Ledo Husby Phillips, Lauren Reich, Katrina Milbocker, and Tania L. Roth. 2020. "Epigenetic consequences of adversity and intervention throughout the lifespan: Implications for public policy and healthcare." *Adversity and Resilience Science* 1 (3):205–16. doi: 10.1007/s42844-020-00015-5.

de Cabo, Rafael, Dan L. Longo, and Mark P. Mattson. 2019. "Effects of intermittent fasting on health, aging, and disease." *New England Journal of Medicine* 381 (26):2541–51. doi: 10.1056/NEJMra1905136.

Gaspard, Ulysse, Mélanie Taziaux, Marie Mawet, Maud Jost, Valérie Gordenne, Herjan J. T. Coelingh Bennink, et al. 2020. "A multicenter, randomized study to select the minimum effective dose of estetrol (E4) in postmenopausal women (E4Relief): part 1. Vasomotor symptoms and overall safety." *Menopause* 27 (8):848–57. doi: 10.1097/gme.0000000000001561.

Monteiro-Junior, Renato Sobral, Paulo de Tarso Maciel-Pinheiro, Eduardo da Matta Mello Portugal, Luiz Felipe da Silva Figueiredo, Rodrigo Terra, et al. 2018. "Effect of exercise on inflammatory profile of older persons: Systematic review and meta-analyses." *Journal of Physical Activity and Health* 15 (1):64–71. doi: 10.1123/jpah.2016-0735.

Robinson, M. M., S. Dasari, A. R. Konopka, M. L. Johnson, S. Manjunatha, R. R. Esponda, et al. 2017. "Enhanced protein translation underlies improved metabolic and physical adaptations to different exercise training modes in young and old humans." *Cell Metabolism* 25 (3):581–92. doi: 10.1016/j.cmet.2017.02.009.

Sparkman, Nathan L., and Rodney W. Johnson. 2008. "Neuroinflammation associated with aging sensitizes the brain to the effects of infection or stress." *Neuroimmunomodulation* 15 (4–6):323–30. doi: 10.1159/000156474.

Uchoa, Mariana F., V. Alexandra Moser, and Christian J. Pike. 2016. "Interactions between inflammation, sex steroids, and Alzheimer's disease risk factors." *Frontiers in Neuroendocrinology* 43:60–82. doi: 10.1016/j.yfrne.2016.09.001.

Vamvakopoulos, N. C., and G. P. Chrousos. 1993. "Evidence of direct estrogenic regulation of human corticotropin-releasing hormone gene expression. Potential implications for the sexual dimorphism of the stress response and immune/inflammatory reaction." *Journal of Clinical Investigation* 92 (4):1896–902. doi: 10.1172/jci116782.

Index

About the Author

Louann Brizendine, MD is the Lynne and Marc Benioff Endowed Chair in Clinical Psychiatry at the University of California, San Francisco, founder of UCSF's Women's Mood and Hormone Clinic, and *New York Times* bestselling author of *The Female Brain* and *The Male Brain*. She lives in Sausalito, California, with her husband, Samuel Barondes.

Also by bestselling author
LOUANN BRIZENDINE, MD

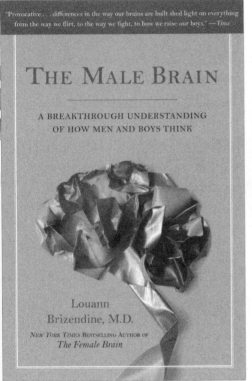

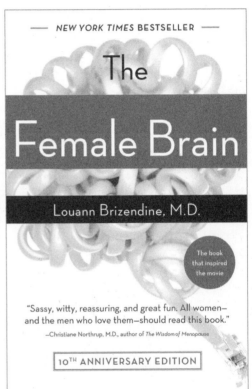

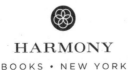